MENTAL TOUGHNESS

Master your mind, change your mental models and boost your confidence (stoicism)

This Book includes:

Self Discipline for Success

Self Esteem Workbook

Improve Your Social Skills

Jack Gilman

Table of Contents

Improve Your Social Skills

Self Discipline for success

A complete blueprint for changing your models and habits, boosting your mental toughness and taking emotional control to achieve your goals and get everything you want.

Jack Gilman

Introduction

Self-discipline is one of the most useful and vital skills that everyone will benefit from having. This skill is crucial in pretty much every area of a person's life. Although most people know how important this skill is, not many take the time to practice strengthening it. The common belief regarding self-discipline is living a strict and limited lifestyle while being harsh to oneself. However, self-discipline just means self-control and building the inner strength to control yourself, your behavior, and your reactions.

Self-discipline is the power that a person has in order to be able to stick with their decisions and to follow them through without changing their minds. This is one of the most important conditions before one can achieve their goals. Having self-discipline allows people to persevere with their decisions and continues to plan to accomplish their goals. Self-discipline can also be known as inner strength, which helps people overcome obstacles like laziness, procrastination, and even addiction.

One of the main traits of self-discipline is the ability to deny instant gratification and pleasure in return for greater gain, which requires a person to put in effort and time to achieve. Most people know that self-discipline is one of the most crucial components when it comes to success. Here is how self-discipline expresses itself:

- Self-control

- Perseverance

- The ability to not give up even when faced with obstacles and failure

- The ability to resist temptations or distractions

- The ability to keep trying until you accomplish the goal you've set

Life is full of challenges and problems—this is one of the inevitable things that we have to accept. When a person is faced with obstacles, they have to act with perseverance and persistence in order to stay on track with their journey to success and achievement. In order to rise above these obstacles, you will require self-discipline. If a person possesses self-discipline, it often leads to building other positive components of a person, such as their self-confidence and self-esteem. Having a good balance of these components in a person's life leads to higher happiness and satisfaction. However, if a person lacks self-discipline, it often leads to negative things like failure, health, loss, obesity, relationship problems, and many other undesirable things. Self-discipline is a useful skill that people can learn to overcome negative habits, such as eating disorders, addictions, smoking, and drinking. Everyone requires it in order to make themselves exercise, develop new skills, study, improve themselves, meditate, and even grow spiritually. Like we mentioned above, many people understand all the benefits of having strong self-discipline, but not many actually do the work to develop and strengthen it. Self-discipline is a skill just like any other—you have the ability to strengthen it as long as you keep practicing it. You can specifically focus on building your self-discipline skills through the use of exercises and training.

So why is self-discipline so important and helpful to most people? Here are all the possible things that self-discipline can help a person with:

- Fulfilling the promises that a person makes to themselves or other people

- Avoiding acting rashly or impulsively

- Continuing to work on goals even after the initial surge of enthusiasm is gone

- Overcoming procrastination and laziness

- Continuing to work on your diet and constantly fighting the urge to eat unhealthy foods

- Going to the gym or getting exercise despite your mind telling you to stay home and watch TV instead

- Waking up early in the morning

- Overcoming bad habits like watching too much TV

- Meditating regularly

- Starting to read a book and finishing it

For a person to strengthen their self-discipline, they may find it easier if they understand a few of its fundamental qualities. You must:

- Understand the importance of self-discipline in your life.

- Be aware of what your undisciplined behavior is, as well as what consequences it brings. When this awareness is increased, you will be more motivated to change your life.

- Try to behave and act in accordance with the decisions or goals you make despite the tendency to procrastinate, desire to give up, and general laziness.

- Strengthen your self-discipline, even if it's weak, by simply exercising your self-discipline muscle, which you can practice anywhere and anytime.

So, you're probably wondering, "What can I achieve through strengthening self-discipline?" You can achieve most of the goals you set for yourself if your mindset is there. Throughout this book, we will be learning about different ways through which you can achieve self-discipline. Popular techniques include visualization and meditation. These are techniques that people use to envision themselves—achieving the goals and success that they want in life. By being able to picture what they want, people have achieved goals that they never thought were possible just by altering their mindset and overcoming bad habits. People like athletes and entrepreneurs all rely heavily on their self-discipline ability in order to achieve the success that they want. Those that are in industries where their successes highly rely on their ability to perform tend to naturally showcase better self-discipline behavior due to having more practice from exercising it every day. For example, people in sales tend to showcase more self-discipline than other occupations because of the targets that they must meet. People within the sales industry are normally hired due to their motivation to make money. Due to this motivation, they likely have a goal or target in mind for how much they want to sell within a certain time frame. By having a defined goal, they are driven to do everything they can to reach it and is constantly overcoming obstacles like instant gratification and laziness. If a person is constantly overcoming those obstacles every day, those obstacles slowly start to feel like they aren't there anymore. *That's* when self-discipline becomes a habit. This is the goal that I want us to get to throughout this book.

In this book, you will learn everything about the psychology behind self-discipline, the benefits and drawbacks of strengthening self-discipline, why self-discipline is the key to success, ten steps that a person needs to take to achieve self-discipline, extensive tips and habits to help build self-discipline, challenges you will come across while you are building self-discipline, visualization and meditation techniques to grow self-discipline, examples of famous people who used self-discipline to achieve success, and finally, an assessment to help determine your level of self-discipline. The way that this book is structured is to help you learn what self-discipline actually is and how it manifests within us before we get into the practical exercises. You will be learning all the behind-the-scenes effects and benefits that self-discipline will bring and some challenges that you will face along the way. You will be learning different techniques and hearing some stories of successful people who used self-discipline to accomplish their goals. Once you have learned the foundation of self-discipline, its benefits, its challenges, and its techniques, then you will move on to completing some self-discipline exercises and beginning to apply them in your life. This book is written simply so that everyone, no matter their education or experience level, would be able to benefit from reading it.

One of the most important things to keep in mind while reading this book is to have an open mind. Some of the topics or ideas that we will be talking about may seem cliché or stereotypical on the outside, but they are provided to you for a reason. Some people may think that techniques like meditation and visualization are 'airy-fairy' and won't work for them because they aren't 'that person.' However, these techniques have been thoroughly studied by multiple professionals in the field of psychology. There are numerous published books, studies, and articles that have found a plethora of evidence that supports the effectiveness of these techniques. Also, you've got nothing to lose! Take these techniques seriously and try to exercise them in your life. Many people tend just to finish reading a book but don't actually begin any of the exercises or build the mindsets that are recommended. By applying the information that you have learned in this book in your daily life, *that* is when you will start achieving the goals that you have set for yourself.

Hence, no matter how young or old, how inexperienced or experienced, or what education level you have, this book will be able to help you strengthen your self-discipline so that you can utilize it in your daily life to achieve the things that you want to achieve. They don't have to be huge goals like building your own billion-dollar company, but you can use it to start achieving some little things that you want in life. This can be quitting smoking, eating healthier, or completing a personal project that's important to you. Regardless of who you are and what you want to accomplish, the basis of self-discipline is the same for everyone. This book will help you understand everything you need to know about self-discipline, as well as the benefits and challenges that it brings—and I will provide you with a step-by-step process on how you can achieve self-discipline, along with some practical exercises that you can use to strengthen it.

So, let's get to it! We will dive into the first chapter, which is learning about the psychology behind self-discipline.

Chapter 1: The Psychology Behind Self-Discipline

Understanding the psychology behind self-discipline is extremely crucial, as it will help you learn what the driving factors are behind it. One of the main factors that drive self-discipline is willpower. A common belief in people is that they think they can change their lives for the better if they simply could just have more willpower. If people had more willpower, everyone would be able to save responsibly for retirement, exercise regularly, stop procrastinating, avoid alcohol and drugs, and achieve all kinds of their noble goals. One survey that studied all Americans and their annual stress found that most of the participants reported that lacking willpower is the number one reason for not following the changes that they want for themselves.

Willpower

In the survey that we just mentioned, it was reported that the biggest obstacle when it comes to people achieving change was the lack of willpower. Even though many people often place blame upon the scarcity of their willpower for their unhealthy choices, they are still grasping on to the hope of being able to achieve it one day. Most people in this study also reported that they think willpower is something that can be taught and learned. They are absolutely correct. Some research recently has discovered many ways of how willpower can be strengthened with training and practice. On the contrary, some participants in the survey expressed that they think they would have more willpower if they had more free time to spare. However, the concept of willpower isn't something that increases automatically if a person has more time in their day. Thus, that leads me to the next question—how can people resist when they are faced with temptation? Over the last several years, many discoveries were made about how willpower works by scientists all over the world. We will dive a little deeper into what our current understanding of willpower is.

Weak willpower isn't the only reason for a person to fail at achieving their goals. Psychologists in the field of willpower have built three crucial components when it comes to achieving goals. They said that you first need to set a clear goal and then establish the motivation for change. They said the second component was to monitor your behavior in regard to that goal. Willpower itself is the third and final component. If your goal is like the following—stop smoking, get fit, study more, or stop wasting time on the internet. Willpower is an important concept to understand if you are looking to achieve any of those goals.

The bottom line of willpower is the ability to achieve long-term goals by resisting temporary temptations and urges. Here are several reasons why this is beneficial. Over the course of a regular school year, psychologists performed a study that examined the self-control in a class of eighth-grade students. The researchers in this study performed an initial assessment of the self-discipline within the students by getting them, their parents, and their teachers to fill out a questionnaire. They took it one step further and gave these students the task of deciding whether they want to receive $1 right away or $2 if they waited a week. At the end of the study, the results pointed to the fact that the students that had better test scores, better school attendance, better grades, and had a higher chance of being admitted to competitive high school programs all ranked high on the self-discipline assessment. These researchers found that self-discipline played a bigger role than IQ when it came to predict academic success. Other studies have found similar evidence. In a different study, researchers asked a group of undergraduate university students to fill out self-discipline questionnaires that will be used to assess their self-control. These researchers developed a scale that helped score the students in relation to the strength of their willpower. They found that the students that had higher self-esteem, better relationship skills, higher GPA, and less alcohol or drug abuse all had the highest self-control scores from the questionnaire.

Another study found that the benefits of willpower tend to be relevant well past university years. This self-control study was conducted in a group of 1000 people who had been tracked since birth to the age of 32. This is a long-term study in New Zealand, where they wanted to learn more about the effects of self-control well into adulthood. They found that the people who had high self-control during their childhood grew up into adults that had better mental and physical health. They also had fewer substance abuse problems, criminal convictions, better financial security, and better money-saving habits. These patterns were proven even after the researchers had adjusted external influences such as socioeconomic factors, general intelligence, and these people's home lives. These findings prove why willpower is extremely important in almost all areas of a person's life.

Now that you have learned the importance of willpower and the role it plays in multiple stages of a person's life, let's define it a little further. There are many other names used for willpower that is used interchangeably. This includes drive, determination, self-control, resolve, and self-discipline. Some psychologists will characterize willpower in even more specific ways. Some define willpower to be:

- The capacity to overcome unwanted impulses, feelings, or thoughts

- The ability to resist temporary urges, temptation and delay instant gratification in order to achieve goals that are more long-term

- The effortful and conscious regulation of oneself

- The ability to engage a "cool" cognitive system of behavior rather than a "hot" emotional system

- A limited resource that has the capability to be depleted

Delaying Gratification

Over 40 years ago, a famous psychologist studied self-control within children using a simple and effective test. You may have seen this study used before in modern-day experiments. His experiment is called the "marshmallow test." This test has become extremely famous over the years as it laid the groundwork and then paved the way for modern studies of self-control.

This psychologist and his colleagues began the test by showing a plate of marshmallows to a child at the preschool age. Then, the psychologist lets the child know that he had to go outside for a few moments and that he would let the child make a very simple decision. If the child could wait until the psychologist came back into the room, she could have two marshmallows. If the child could not or doesn't want to wait, then she can ring the bell, which then the psychologist would come back to the room right away, but then, she would only get to have one marshmallow.

Willpower can be defined as simple as the ability for a person to delay instant gratification. Children who have high self-control are able to give up the immediate gratification of eating a marshmallow so that they can be able to eat two of them at a later time. People who have quit smoking do sacrifice the satisfaction of one cigarette in hopes of having better health and lower the risk of cancer in the future. Shoppers fight the urge to spend money at a mall so they can save their money for their future retirement. You probably get the point here.

This marshmallow experiment actually helped the researchers develop a framework that explains people's ability to resist or delay instant gratification. He proposed a system that he calls "hot and cool" in order to explain whether willpower will succeed or fail. The 'cool' system is naturally a cognitive one. It means that it is a thinking system that uses knowledge about feelings, sensations, goals, and actions that remind oneself, for example, why the marshmallow shouldn't be eaten. The cool system is very reflective, while the hot system is more emotional and impulsive. The hot system is responsible for quick and reflex-based responses to specific triggers, for example, eating the single marshmallow without thinking about the long-term ramifications. To put this in layman's terms, if this framework were a cartoon, the hot system would be the devil, and the cool system would be the angel on your shoulder.

When somebody's willpower fails, their hot system essentially overrides their cool system, which leads them to make impulsive actions. However, some people are more or less affected by the hot system triggers. That susceptibility to emotional responses plays a big role in influencing a person's behavior throughout life. The same researcher discovered that when he revisited his experiment with the children that had now grown up into adolescents, he found that the teenagers who were able to wait longer to have two marshmallows when they were children were more likely to have higher SAT grades and their parents were more likely to rate them of having better ability to handle stress, plan, respond to reason and exhibit self-control in frustrating situations and could concentrate better without being easily distracted.

Funnily enough, the marshmallow study didn't end there. A few other researchers tracked down almost 60 people who are now middle-aged, who had previously been a part of the marshmallow experiment as young children. These psychologists proceeded to test the participants' willpower strength using a task that's been proven to prove self-control within adults. Surprisingly, the participants' various willpower strengths had been very consistent over the last 40 years. Overall, they found that the children who were not successful in resisting the first marshmallow did poorly on the self-control tasks as an adult and that their hot stimuli seem to be consistent throughout their lifetime. They also began to study brain activity in some of the participants by using magnetic resonance technology. When these participants were presented with tempting stimuli, those who had low willpower exhibited brain patterns that were very different from the brain patterns of those that had strong willpower. They discovered that the prefrontal cortex (this is the region of the brain that controls choice-making functions) was more active in the participants who had stronger willpower and the ventral striatum (an area of the brain that is focused on processing rewards and desires) showed increased activity in the participants who had weaker willpower.

Is Willpower a Limited Resource?

The hot-cold framework does a great job of explaining people's ability to delay gratification, but there is another theory that is called 'willpower depletion' that has emerged in recent years to explain what happens to people after they have resisted multiple temptations. Everyone exerts willpower every day in one form or another. People resist to surf the web or go on social media instead of finishing their work report. They may choose a salad when they are craving a slice of pizza. They may hold their tongue rather than make a snide remark. Recent growing research indicates that resisting temptations takes a mental toll on a person repeatedly. Some people describe willpower as a muscle that can get tired if overused.

The earliest discoveries of this concept came from a study that was conducted in Germany. The researcher brought participants into a room that smelled like fresh-baked cookies. The participants sat down at the table that held a bowl of radishes and a plate of those freshly baked cookies. The researchers asked some of the participants to taste those cookies while the others were asked to try the radishes. After this, the participants were assigned to complete a difficult geometric puzzle in 30 minutes. The researchers found that the participants who had to eat the radishes (therefore resisting the urge to eat the cookies) took 8 minutes to give up on the puzzle while the participants who got to eat the cookies tried to complete the puzzle for 19 minutes. The evidence here seems as if the people who used their willpower to resist eating the cookies drained their resources for future situations.

In the late 90s, this research was published, and since then, numerous other studies have begun looking into willpower depletion or otherwise known as ego depletion. One study, for example, the participants were asked to hold back and suppress any feelings they had while they watched an emotional film. These participants then participated in a physical stamina test but gave up sooner than the participants who watched the movie and reacted normally without any suppression.

Depleting willpower is very common today. You have probably tried to make yourself be diplomatic when you are dealing with an aggravating customer or forced to fake happiness when your in-laws come to stay with you for an extended period. You must have realized that certain social interacts demand the use of willpower. There is also existing research that has proven that people interacting with others and maintaining relationships often is a high reducer of willpower.

Willpower depletion is not solely just a simple case of feeling tired. During another study by the same researcher, she had the participants in her study go through a whole day of sleep deprivation and then asked them to watch a movie but to suppress their emotions and reactions during it. She then proceeded to test the strength of the participant's self-control and found that those participants who didn't get sleep were not much more likely to be depleted of willpower compared to those who got a full night's sleep.

So, if willpower isn't related to physical fatigue, then what exactly is it? Research studies recently have discovered a few different mechanisms that are possibly responsible for willpower depletion, some that were at the biological level. The researchers found that the people whose willpower became depleted after completing self-control tasks showed lowered activity in the region of their brain that controlled cognition. When willpower is being tested, a person's brain may begin to function differently.

Some other evidence indicates that people who have depleted willpower might be on low on fuel quite literally. Since the brain is an organ requiring high amounts of energy that is powered by glucose, certain professionals suggested that the cells in the brain that are responsible for maintaining a person's self-control do use up glucose quicker than it is being replenished. They performed a study with dogs where the dogs that were obedient and were asked to resist temptation showed lower blood glucose levels compared to the dogs that did not need to use self-control.

They found similar patterns in humans during scientific studies. The people who needed to use willpower in tasks were tested to have lower glucose levels compared to the participants that weren't asked to utilize their willpower. Moreover, replenishing glucose levels tend to help reboot a depleted willpower source in individuals that were depleted while drinking a sugar-free drink did not.

However, there is still evidence that suggests that the depletion of willpower can be maintained by a person's attitudes and beliefs. Different research and other colleagues found out that the people who felt the need to use their willpower (usually in order to please other people) were found to be more easily depleted compared to the people who are driven by their own desires and goals. These researchers, therefore, suggested that the people who are in better touch with themselves may be better off in life compared to the people who are often people-pleasing.

Some other researchers also studied how the effects of mood could affect a person's willpower. A study that took place in 2010 discovered that the group of people who believed that willpower is a resource that is limited were more likely to have willpower depletion. However, the group of people that did not believe that willpower can be depleted didn't show any symptoms or signs of willpower exhaustion after using their self-control. During the next stage of the same study, the psychologists manipulated the participants' subconscious beliefs by getting them to fill out a biased questionnaire unknowingly. The group that was manipulated to believe that willpower is for a fact a limited resource exhibited symptoms of willpower depletion/exhaustion, while the group that believed that willpower was not expendable didn't show any signs of declining self-control.

So, at the end of all this evidence and discussion, do you think willpower is a limited resource? Many ideas point to evidence that supports both spectrums of this answer. They argued that willpower depletion in the early stages could be buggered by factors such as belief and mood. However, more research is definitely required for us to explore how moods, attitudes, and beliefs might be affecting a person's ability to resist temptation.

Healthy Behaviors and Willpower

A person makes decisions every day in order to resist urges and gratification so that they can seek a healthier and happy long-term life. This could be in the form of refusing another portion of fries, forcing yourself to go work out, denying another round of alcoholic drinks, or overcoming the temptation to skip early morning meetings. Willpower within everyone is being tested on a constant basis.

Lack of willpower is often known as the main obstacle to people's ability to maintain a healthy weight and physique. A lot of research actually supports this idea. A study found that children that had better self-control had less likelihood of becoming overweight when they grew up into their adolescence years due to their ability to delay gratification and control their urges.

However, just like we talked about earlier, resisting those urges may diminish a person's willpower to resist the next temptation. A researcher proved this in a study where they offered students that were currently dieting some ice cream after watching a sad movie. Some of the participants were asked to watch the movie like any other normal day while the other group was asked not to show any reactions or emotions, which is a task that requires self-control. The psychologists discovered that the participants who had to use their self-control to withhold their emotions and reactions indulged in more ice cream compared to the participants who could watch the movie normally and react as they'd like.

A lot of people often place most of the blame on their bad moods for causing their 'emotional eating.' However, that study found that the participants' emotional states were not the cause of the amount of ice cream that they consumed. In layman's terms, the depletion of willpower had more significance than a person's mood when it comes to determining how much ice cream the participants ate.

We must keep in mind that the reason behind why someone is on a diet will also play a role in willpower depletion. As we had just discussed, researchers found that people's attitudes and inner beliefs may create a buffer for them in terms of the effects of willpower depletion. In a further example that this based on this theory, the researchers asked participants to resist the temptation of eating cookies that were placed in front of them. He then tested the participant's strength of self-control by getting them to squeeze an exercise handgrip until they couldn't anymore He discovered through this exercise that the people who refused to eat the cookies for their own reasons (such as finding enjoyment in resisting treats) showed better control in this physical test compared to the ones who refused the cookies for reasons that were external (wanting to impress the experimenter).

At this point, it is obvious that willpower is a required component when it comes to eating healthy. If a person is living in a surrounding where there were plenty of unhealthy but delicious food options, the action of resisting temptation is more likely to deplete willpower and even making it difficult for highly motivated healthy eaters. Since the behaviors of overeating are very complex, the role of willpower is argumentative when it comes to discussions for obesity treatments.

Some of the experts in the field of willpower believe that using self-control and personal choices causes people to be stigmatized, which makes them unlikely to be motivated to lose weight. Many dieticians advise against using willpower as a tool and argue that dieters should be focusing on lowering the effect that their environment will have on their eating habits and behavior. Ultimately, when it comes to the world we live in today, resisting the temptation to eat unhealthily can be a hard challenge. We are constantly exposed to ads for delicious high-calorie foods. Cheap and fast processed foods are available at our fingertips 24/7 and are less expensive compared to healthier options. A person's willpower and the environment that they live in do play a big role in people's choices when it relates to food. Having a better understanding of both elements will help individuals and dieticians that are battling obesity.

Not only does willpower play a role in eating healthy, but it also plays a role in the use and possible abuse of alcohol, tobacco, and drugs. Children who have developed self-control may avoid substance abuse in their adulthood and teenage years. Researchers in this field studied the self-control of adolescents as they moved from sixth grade to eleventh grade.

They discovered that the kids who had problems with self-control in the sixth grade, such as not speaking in turn during class, had more likelihood of using tobacco, marijuana, and alcohol as high school students.

This may not come as surprising, but willpower also plays a significant role in curbing alcohol abuse and usage. In another study, a researcher discovered that people who drank socially very often that used their willpower during the lab proceeded to go out and consume more alcohol compared to the other participants who didn't use their willpower stockpile. In a different study, the researcher found that the social drinkers who had used a lot of their self-control that day were more likely to infringe on the drinking limits that they created for themselves. This finding shows evidence that exerting self-control excessively in one situation can cripple a person's ability to fight off other temptations in different parts of their life.

We are talking a lot about willpower because understanding the role that it plays is very important for developing effective treatments and plan to battle serious issues like addictions to help guide people in making healthier choices for themselves. Willpower research offers people lots of suggestions on how to stick with healthy behaviors.

The Role of Willpower in Relation to Financial Decision-Making

The temptation of consuming in materialistic things like new shoes or a new car is a test of willpower that we have all experienced. Just like how unhealthy food options have become plentiful, the opportunities for impulse spending has grown as well. ATMs are on every corner, and the rise of shopping online only allows a person to spend all their money without even having to leave the comfort of their couch. Willpower depletion affects people's ability to choose healthier lifestyle options and also affects their purchasing behavior.

Professors from the University of Minnesota did a study that focused on impulse buying and willpower depletion. They showed the participants a silent movie with a series of words that appeared on the bottom of the screen. A group of those participants was asked not to pay attention to those words, which was a task that required the use of self-control. After the movie, the participants were asked to look through a catalog with products like cars and watches, and they wrote down the money amount that they were willing to pay for every single item. The participants that used self-control during the movie were willing to spend more money, about $30,000, while the participants who didn't deplete their willpower were willing to spend approximately $23,000.

In the next experiment, the researchers tested the spending behavior of the participants by showing them the opportunity to buy lower-cost objects like cups and decorative stickers. The group that had done self-control in the previous experiment expressed that they felt a higher temptation to buy those items. In fact, they purchased more items and spent more money compared to the participants who hadn't done the self-control exercise.

The task of making financial decisions can be much harder for people that are impoverished. Researchers conducted various studies in India to explore the relationship between poverty and willpower strength. In one study, this researcher visited two different Villages—one that was poor and one that was richer. The researcher offered people an opportunity to buy a luxury brand name soap at an extremely discounted price tag. This item was a great deal in terms of cost, but it still showed that people who live in poverty had difficulty making financial decisions as such.

The participants in the study were told to squeeze a handgrip made for exercise, which is a popular test of strength regarding self-control, before and after the soap was offered to be purchased. The researcher found that the participants who had more money exercised the handgrip for the same amount of time prior and subsequent to the opportunity to buy that soap. However, they found that poor participants squeezed the handgrip for a smaller amount of time after making a purchasing decision. Their willpower was depleted, and the researcher had concluded that it was run down by the difficulty of making that financial decision.

This research may sound depressing, but there is a silver lining. If impoverished people have a higher chance of using up their willpower, then it could possibly mean that lowering the number of hard decisions that they have to make every day to help prevent the depletion of willpower will give them the ability to make future decisions. A different researcher studied this effect amongst thanking customers in Southeast Asia. They offered customers the opportunity to open a savings account, but it comes with a catch. These customers would only be able to withdraw their funds after reaching a targeted saving goal or target date that they have decided for themselves. A year later, the participants that signed up for these accounts saved 82% more than the participants who had not opened the special savings account. When the decision to save money or spend money is taken away, it helps customers avoid failing at self-control.

All of this evidence shows that the people who are in the lower end of the socioeconomic spectrum are more likely to deplete their self-control resources. It's not that people who don't have money have less willpower than rich people; rather, the people that are living in poverty must make more willpower draining decisions. This means that every decision they make—whether it is as simple as buying soap—will require self-control, which, therefore, dips into their limited resources of willpower.

Improving Self-Control

A ton of research has been developed recently in order to explain the numerous elements of willpower. Many professionals that study this area of self-control to this with one goal on their mind. They are about these types of questions: If willpower is a limited resource, what can we do to conserve it? How can we strengthen willpower?

One effective tactic for maintaining willpower is simply to avoid temptation. In the marshmallow study, children were given a choice of being allowed to eat one marshmallow right away or having to wait an undefined period to have the opportunity to eat two marshmallows. They found that the kids who started at the marshmallows during the whole time were found to be less likely to resist the food compared to the kids who shut their eyes and refused to look, looked away, or created a distraction for themselves. The technique of out of sight, out of mind, works with adults as well. In a recent study, researchers found that office workers who kept unhealthy snacks, such as candy in their desk drawers, consumed it less compared to when they would put the candy on top of their desks at eye level.

A technique called "implementation intention" is another helpful tactic that helps improve willpower. These intentions are usually in the form of "if-then" statements that aid people in planning for situations that are likely to disrupt their goals. For instance, a person that is monitoring their consumption of alcohol may tell themselves before entering a drinking part that is anybody offers them an alcoholic drink, then they will request a plain soda with lime. Research has found that amongst adults and adolescents, implementing solutions will increase self-control, even if people already had their willpower depleted by other tasks. People that have a plan ahead of time allows them to easily make decisions at the moment without needing to draw upon their bank of willpower resources.

This research suggests that people who have a bank of willpower that is limited raises a few troubling questions. Are people destined to fail if they are being faced with too many temptations? The answer is not necessarily. Many psychologists have the belief that a person's willpower cannot be ever used up completely. Instead, people often have stored some backup willpower that is being saved for future demands. Those reserves are only available for the right type of motivation, allowing them to accomplish things even when their willpower has seemingly run out.

In order to demonstrate this idea, a researcher further found out that individuals who had their willpower used up 'completely' continued to be able to accomplish self-control tasks when they were being told that they would be compensated well for their actions or if their actions would bring benefit to other people. He concluded that having high motivation can overcome weaken self-control.

Willpower can also be controlled in the first place to be less vulnerable to being completely depleted. Psychologists often use an analogy to describe willpower as being similar to a muscle that will tire out after a long duration of the exercise. However, there is another element to this analogy. Although muscles will tire due to exercise during the short-term, they become stronger when regularly exercised over the long term.

Just like physical exercise, self-control can become stronger when a person exercises willpower.

According to one of the earlier experiments that supports the idea above, the researchers asked participants in the study to follow a two-week guide to improve their moods, track their food intake, or improve their physical posture. Compared to the group that didn't need to exercise self-control, the participants who had to use their willpower by performing heavy willpower exercises were not as vulnerable to the depletion of self-control in a follow-up study. In another set of research, this researcher found that smokers who exercised willpower for two weeks by avoiding sweet foods or regularly squeezing an exercise handgrip, found more success when it comes to not smoking than other participants who performed two weeks of tasks that didn't require any self-control.

Other researchers have also discovered that using your willpower muscles can help a person increase the strength of their self-control over a period of time. Some researchers in Australia did a study where they assigned participants to a physical exercise program that lasted two months—this is a willpower-required routine. In the conclusion of this program, the participants that finished it scored better when measuring self-control compared to the other participants who were not assigned the exercise program. The participants that did the program were also reported to have been smoking less, eating healthier food, drinking less alcohol, improving their study habits, and monitoring their spending habits more carefully. Regular exercise of a person's willpower using physical exercise seem to have led to an increase of willpower in components of their daily lives.

The research findings regarding how glucose levels are tied to willpower depletion suggest a conceivable solution. A person that is maintains their blood sugar by eating regularly and often may help their brain replenish their storage of willpower. Those who are dieting aim to preserve their willpower, while calorie reduction may be more effective by eating frequent and small meals compared to skipping out on entire meals like lunch or dinner.

All this evidence, founded from studies of the depletion of willpower, proposes that people making resolutions for the new year is the worst approach possible. If a person is running low on willpower in one specific area, it often reduces their willpower in all of the other areas. Focusing on one goal at a time makes more sense. In other words, don't try to get into a healthy diet right away, quit smoking, and start a new workout plan all at the same time. A much better technique is to complete goals one by one. Once you have one single good habit nailed, people no longer need to use their supply of willpower to maintain that behavior. Habits that are healthy will eventually become a part of a person's daily routine and would not need to use the energy of decision-making at all.

There are still many questions regarding the nature of willpower that needs to be answered by future research. However, it seems like if somebody has clear goals, good self-monitoring, and does a little bit of practice, they can train their self-control to be strong when faced with temptation.

Chapter 2: Benefits and Drawbacks of Strengthening Self-Discipline

In the last chapter, you learned about all the research that went behind studying willpower, which is a huge component of self-discipline. You learned that people's willpower resources had the ability to be depleted, but you also learned that having a positive mindset can create a buffer for which willpower is depleted. In this chapter, you will learn about the benefits that having strong self-discipline can bring. We will be discussing five main benefits that self-discipline can add to your life. In addition, we will also learn about what causes someone to have low self-discipline. In the previous chapter, we learned that willpower has the ability to affect all aspects of a person's life positively. Similarly, the lack of self-discipline can also negatively affect each aspect of a person's life.

Benefits of Having Self-Discipline

When a person has strong self-discipline, it leads to higher self-regard, inner strength, self-assurance, and ultimately, satisfaction and happiness. It leads to better outcomes in every area of a person's life. The following benefits of self-discipline are ones that may not automatically come to mind.

Benefit #1: Self-Discipline Creates Inner Strength and Character

According to a famous psychology book, there was an important statement that the author wrote. He stated that everyone is the person that they wish to be. All that is stopping you from behaving in the manner that you want to behave is your emotional mind. Let's think about that for a second. Although you may be a very kind and caring person, if you tend to lose your temper easily, other people may see you as a hothead or an angry person. In this example, you don't necessarily need to change who you are as a person. Instead, you need to change the way you behave. Once you change the way you behave, other people will then see you for the person that you truly are. For example, you already are that kind and caring person, but your short temper is preventing you from showing that personality to the world. Your self-discipline is a tool that can help you to stop acting on your impulses and instead act based on your true character.

Benefit #2: Self-Discipline Allows You to Resist Temptations

As we discussed in chapter one, our modern-day lives are filled to the brim with temptations that can throw people off track and prevent them from achieving their goals. Often, these temptations are temporary, and by exercising willpower, most people can overcome the urge. In our modern workplace, temptations tend to take the form of distractions like checking your phone, a conversation at the water cooler, or scrolling through social media. Those examples are just the tip of the iceberg when it comes to our potential modern-day distractions. When you can recognize what your temptations are, you can place a strategy in order to prevent caving to it. This requires less self-discipline compared to ignoring the temptation with brute mental force. For example, if your coworker locks her phone in the drawer of her desk and refuses to check her phone during the workday. She may make this strategy easier for her by telling all her friends that she does this so that her friends do not expect an immediate response.

As we already learned, temptations also exist in the form of addictions and bad habits. When self-disciplined is coupled with effective strategies, it is a very valuable tool that can be used to overcome most urges in life.

Benefit #3: Stronger Self-Discipline Increases One's Chances of Success

When a goal can be achieved with great ease, some would argue whether it should even be considered a goal or not. Goals require a person to stretch and grow; to improve skills, attitudes, and to improve one's knowledge. When an individual meets those requirements, they improve the quality of their life along with improving their capability to take on larger and harder challenges. Ultimately, goals should be challenging. Everyone will face barriers and obstacles in which they would need to overcome. This is the action that is needed in order to create personal growth. In order to overcome these obstacles and barriers to achieve your goals. It will require a lot of self-discipline and self-belief. A person's ability to persevere and overcome obstacles when faced with difficulty is often the difference between failure and success.

Benefit #4: People with Self-Discipline Build Better Relationships

Take a minute to think about some of the things that you value in a relationship. This could be a friendship, a romantic relationship, or a familial relationship. You may value important things like integrity, dependability, loyalty, and honesty. All these traits require a person to have a strong character. It requires someone who can be true and act true to their values and beliefs, even when it would be easier to fall into temptation. As we already discussed, those with self-discipline are more likely to develop a stronger character. They have a lot of practice in doing the things that they know need to be done, even though they would probably rather be doing something else. Generally, they are a person that most people can count on. They are more effective when it comes to gaining respect and building trust amongst their peers.

Benefit #5: Self-Discipline Makes It More Difficult for a Person to Be Offended

People with more self-discipline tend to be calmer, assured, and more confident. They know who they are as a person and what they believe in. They will always do what they believe to be the right thing. As we mentioned throughout this book, although the task that needs to be done may not be something that they want to do at that very moment in time, the strength of self-discipline demands them to be true to their values and beliefs. One of the major benefits of this behavior of a self-disciplined person is that they can always be confident that they have done their best. If a person knows that they tried their very best and couldn't have done any better, they will be able to hold their heads up high, knowing that any insults or criticism are meaningless. However, this person would also be prepared to listen to any constructive criticism, but negative feedback does not affect them much at all. To maximize the benefits of self-discipline, a person must have goals that are effective in motivating and inspiring them.

Reasons Why People Don't Take More Responsibility

At this point, we've learned that having high self-discipline helps people establish their inner strength and character, enables them to withstand temptation, increases their chance of success, builds better relationships, and has more resistance to feeling offended. We will now discuss some of the causes as to why some people have low self-discipline.

Having low self-discipline, not unlike having high self-discipline, affects people's performance in multiple aspects of their life. This includes the performance at work, school, relationships, sports, and financial well-being.

Lack of self-discipline shows up in all the different things that people do in their lives. Some people make sure that they do the big things in life but end up neglecting the little things. They do this to impress other people who don't know them very well. However, they tend to annoy and disappoint those that are close to them because it shows that they don't care enough about the people that they should be showing respect to. When people choose not to perform certain chores or duties, don't do what they say they would, don't show up for appointments, or don't make themselves presentable for every day, they are showing low self-discipline. So, you may be wondering, why don't we take more responsibility for these everyday obligations? Below are two reasons why:

Attitude

One of the reasons why people don't take more responsibility for everyday obligations is because they don't believe in its importance. Why is this? Why do some people take the time to be considerate, clean, trustworthy, and honest While others believe that those things are important? The answer is their attitude towards themselves, other people, and life itself. The former believes that people, including themselves, and other forms of life, are worth investing their energy, time, resources, and interest into. They can see the importance of Life while the latter have less regard for life and for themselves. All the simply relates to love. When people have a love for life, they tend to respect all components of it. They take the time to appreciate and experience life as if it's a pleasure. Self-discipline comes from the willingness to take care of ourselves, other people, and other types of life. The lack of discipline shows less willingness to respect themselves or other things.

Commitment

The second reason why people don't take more responsibility for everyday obligations is because of the lack of commitment. A person's commitment, enthusiasm, and interest to a task determine the degree to which they can be distracted. When their commitment is very high, very few things have the power to distract them, but if they are doing something that is meaningless to them, their attention is easily distracted. This proves a strong link between self-discipline and commitment. People who have the inability to ignore, control, or bypass thoughts means that they have low self-discipline.

Causes of Low Self-Discipline

By learning the reasons behind why a person does not take more responsibility for everyday obligations, we are ready to learn some of the causes of poor self-discipline.

Cause #1: Lack of Awareness

The primary cause of low self-discipline is a lack of awareness. This component is important specifically to our imagination and thinking. People are unaware of the thoughts that take our attention are actually negative and can damage a person's well-being. These thoughts are fed into the conscious mind by the negative mind power to ensure that people have minimal time to spend just simply just being mindful. If people are aware of the things that are happening within their own minds, they would know that self-discipline is needed to refocus our attention away from the flow of negative thoughts.

Cause #2: Character Weaknesses

Oftentimes, people who have weak character creates poor self-discipline. This includes aspects that have a low level of inner strength, mental toughness, courage, lack of love for other people, an absence of self-love, low interest in self-improvement, apathy, shortage of responsibility, lack of self-reflection, high levels of greed, and the inability to ignore temptations, in general.

If people place more importance on the desires, thoughts, and emotions that harm them more than the actions, thoughts, and people that help them, it will be difficult for them to develop high self-discipline. Each moment comes with a choice that a person has to make. Either it can be something that helps them reach the goals that they have set for themselves, or they can fall into temptation and choose the action that has instant gratification.

Cause #3: Lack of Ambition

Ambition is very effective in creating self-discipline by giving us a reason to work towards our goals, although we might rather be doing something else. However, it has a negative effect on our self-discipline if our ambition is in an honorable, ethical, or fulfilling one. It is obvious that people who lack the ambition to achieve goals in life will have a harder time building strong self-discipline because they don't have a reason to do it. This is why we discussed in chapter one that one of the main steps in developing strong self-discipline is coming up with clear and attainable goals. By coming up with a goal that is realistic, an individual can then create a plan of action that they can then hold themselves accountable to. They also need to continue finding the motivation and ambition to keep them striving towards their goals.

Cause #4: Having Goals That Have Low Importance

People that have goals that aren't that important tend to lack the ambition to achieve them and, therefore, will not be able to practice their self-discipline. If people set goals that looked good on the outside but didn't actually believe that they were necessary, or didn't see them as goals that are important enough to accomplish in the first place, then they may find it very difficult exercise self-discipline in order to put in the work to achieve them. One of the main motivating factors of self-discipline is having a goal that a person is able to stand by or is important to them. By having an important goal, or something that is meaningful to them, they will be able to find the self-discipline needed in order to complete the tasks required in order to achieve their goal.

Cause #5: Laziness

There are many temporary reasons as to why a person is not exhibiting self-discipline to do the things that need to be done. This could be sickness, tiredness, apathy, or something that is more appealing that is immediately available. If you find that these excuses were often occurring when you were trying to complete the task needed to reach a goal, you need to dig deep and find the real reason why you are choosing options that aren't the ones that will help you achieve your goal. Laziness is often the culprit in a lot of cases. The reasons for laziness usually run very deep into an individual's psyche. If a person believes that there is a goal that is worthwhile, they will be motivated to keep working and applying themselves and making the decisions that make sense when it comes to achieving their goal. However, if they don't have any motivation to achieve their goal, it likely means that their goal isn't important enough, or the person has a natural tendency to be lazy and uninterested.

Cause #6: Lack of Self-Respect

Oftentimes, a person who is lacking self-respect doesn't put a lot of effort or importance in achieving personal excellence. They often don't really care what others think about them or whether they are helping out other people in their lives or not. You might be wondering what self-respect has to do with self-discipline. The answer is that it takes self-discipline in order to produce excellent results, to achieve goals, and to help people who require it. When a person doesn't think about their own self-improvement, they tend to focus on other things that bring them pleasure such as instant gratification. They don't necessarily practice self-discipline because they are comfortable in indulging the instant gratification that life throws at them. If a person lacks respect for themselves, they are more likely to indulge in unhealthy conveniences like fast food or shopping impulses that we discussed in chapter one. If a person does have self-respect for themselves, they understand that this instant gratification may bring them joy and pleasure at the moment but does very little in helping them achieve healthy long-term goals.

By the end of this chapter, you have learned the benefits of having high self-discipline, the causes of low self-discipline, and the effects it has on a person when they have low self-discipline. By understanding the psychology behind the concept of self-discipline, willpower, and self-control, a person is more likely to see the importance of having these traits if they are a person that wants to achieve the goals they have in life. I strongly believe that everyone has their own personal goals that they want to accomplish in their life. Those who say they don't may simply be too afraid of failure and hide their fear behind their lies about how they don't have goals rather than coming to terms with the fact that they are scared of failing to achieve their goals. In the next chapter, we will be discussing why self-discipline is often the key to success. All the concepts and examples that you learned in the past two chapters will slowly come together in chapter 3 as you learn why self-discipline is absolutely needed when it comes to a person's ability to find success.

Chapter 3: Why Self-Discipline Is the Key to Success

Many researchers suggest that the single most important thing in a person's ability to become successful is their level of self-discipline. Self-discipline is responsible for helping people stay focused on reaching their goals, gives them the grit that they need to stick with difficult tasks, and allows them to overcome barriers and discomforts as they push themselves to achieve greater things. Let's refresh our memory on the definition of self-discipline. Self-discipline is the ability of a person to control their impulses, reactions, behaviors, and emotions. It allows them to let go of instant gratification in exchange for long-term gain and satisfaction. It's the act of saying no when you really want to say yes. Self-discipline isn't about living a restrictive and boring life without any enjoyment. In fact, it's almost impossible to be 100% self-disciplined in every single area of your life. Rather than trying to be disciplined at everything you do; you can use it to focus on the things that are most important to you. In this chapter, we will be discussing all the reasons why self-discipline is crucial to a person's success. We will be going through multiple reasons as to why this is true, and I will provide you with a few tips that will help increase your self-discipline overall.

People Cannot Achieve Their Goals Without Self-Discipline

People cannot achieve their goals without self-discipline, so make sure that you are supplementing your goals with a self-discipline list. It will help you focus on the tasks and behaviors that you need to perform in order to achieve the goals that you want. For example, one of my goals is to lose 10 pounds by December. My discipline list will include things like avoiding fast food, buying more fruits and vegetables, and making sure to hit the gym at least twice a week. High self-discipline, in this example, would be doing everything on that list without any exception. This does not mean that you cannot reward yourself or take a break from working towards your goals; it simply means that you should get the things done on your list before you indulge in any rewards.

Use a Daily "To-Do" List to Track the Things You Need to Get Done

Make sure you are using a daily to-do list to keep track of all the things that you need to get done in order to achieve your goals. Try to use online tools or just a simple notebook that can help you prioritize and organize. It feels very satisfying to be able to check off items that you've completed, and it will even motivate you to finish other tasks that are on your list just to feel the satisfaction of being able to check off another box. Make sure your to-do list works together with your discipline list to help yourself stay on track. A useful tip to keep in mind when you're feeling unmotivated is to start off with the easiest item on the list just to get the ball rolling. Once you complete one easy task, people normally feel more motivated than before; this will help you get started on the rest of your list. Starting with a harder task May create apprehension about doing it, therefore, start small and work your way up.

Figure Out Which Obstacles Are Holding You Back from Success

Different people have different things that distract them from being able to complete important tasks. For example, a person that is easily distracted by emails and people in their office might have to close their office door as soon as they get into work to get their own tasks done. They may delay any phone calls or meetings unless they're absolutely necessary in order to be able to complete their own set of responsibilities. This holds true for people that may be trying to lose weight. If they know that junk food is their weakness, instead of having to resist the temptation of eating junk food in their house, they can simply get rid of all the junk food in their house so that they don't have access to it. It is important that you minimize and remove all temptations of the distractions that affect you the most when it comes to reaching your most important goals.

Share Your Goals with Other People

For some people, it may be easier to stick with completing a goal when they have made a public commitment to it. The thought of failing to reach a goal in front of other people can be motivation for the person to stick with it. You can also take this one step further and ask those people to hold you accountable as well. If you aren't sharing your goals with anyone, nobody will know if you have been slacking off from it. When nobody is there to hold you accountable, you will likely be less motivated to keep doing it since nobody will know if you did fail at it.

Use External and Internal Sources of Motivation

There is a saying that goes, "Don't do it for others; do it for yourself." However, some people find that they are much more disciplined when they know that their impulses, emotions, behaviors, and actions affect other people. Contrary to popular belief, it's alright to use external sources to help your motivation. In fact, sometimes, motivation coming from external sources is more powerful than internal motivation. Find the purpose that's beyond yourself that is important to you in order to help give you a higher chance of success.

Discipline Is Created by Creating Habits

We talked about this in the earlier chapter about how, when something becomes a habit, you no longer need to draw from your willpower bank to get yourself to do it. For example, if a person's goal was to do more exercise, they should make a commitment to work out for at least 20 minutes per day for a whole month. They will be able to see the benefits of regular exercise if they are able to stick with it. Once they see the benefit, they will have more motivation to keep doing it, and soon it becomes a habit where if this person does not do at least 20 minutes of exercise a day, they don't feel good physically. This way, they will no longer need to draw from their bank of self-control, but instead, exercising for them will naturally come since it has become a habit of theirs.

Stop Making Excuses

Don't procrastinate or wait for tomorrow—do it *now*. If you fall off the wagon, that's okay. Start over immediately. Stop telling yourself that something is too hard or that there's something that you cannot change. Don't blame other people for the circumstances that you are in. Making excuses is the Kryptonite of self-discipline. Achieve a mindset that is more about, "I can do this" rather than, "I'll do it tomorrow."

Chapter 4: Ten Steps to Achieve Self-Discipline

At this point in the book, you should have a good understanding of what self-discipline is, as well as the benefits that it brings—and you should now be ready for steps that you can take to achieve it. Everyone faces difficult decisions when they are presented with temptations that are hard to resist. A person that is looking to eat healthier may struggle with their self-discipline when they are offered a hot fudge sundae. A person who is looking to gain some muscle mass may face a temptation of wanting to sleep in rather than going to the gym. People that have stronger self-control often spend less time thinking about whether to indulge in temptations that are bad for their health or not. Instead, they are able to make better decisions for themselves more easily. They don't let feelings or impulses affect their decision-making. They are always able to make level-headed decisions. As a result of this, they feel more satisfied with their life, as they are able to achieve more goals.

There are things that you can do in order to learn self-discipline and tap into your willpower source in order to live a happier life. Below are ten steps that you should follow in order to master your self-discipline.

Step 1: Know Your Weaknesses

Everyone has their own set of weaknesses. They could range from a certain type of food like chocolate, or it can be a social media app like Instagram, or it can even be the latest addictive video game. Regardless of what it is, it has a similar effect on everyone.

The first step to mastering your self-discipline is to acknowledge your shortcomings, no matter what they might be. People often try to pretend that their weaknesses don't exist in order to portray themselves as a strong person. This is extremely ineffective when it comes to self-discipline. The purpose of acknowledging your weaknesses is not to make yourself feel bad. Instead, it helps you to recognize what they are—and this will help you to plan in advance to overcome them. Acknowledge your flaws—it is impossible to overcome them until you do this.

Step 2: Remove Your Temptations

Once you have acknowledged your weaknesses, you can now move on to step two, which is to remove your temptations. Just like we mentioned in step one, everyone has their own set of weaknesses, and it can range from small things like an unhealthy snack all the way to something that hinders your productivity, like playing a video game for hours on end. By understanding what your weaknesses are, you can make accommodations for yourself that will help remove some of those temptations.

For example, if somebody is looking to lose weight and get fit at the gym, but they know that their weakness is that they always eat chocolate after dinner every night. Their temptation removal, in this case, would be not to buy any more chocolate that they keep around in their home. By not having chocolate in the home, they would be unable to fall into the temptation of eating it, which will hinder their progress of getting fit. However, this does not mean that they will never be able to eat chocolate again. This only means that they can indulge in their favorite snacks when they have achieved a certain portion of their goal. Rewarding oneself is important to self-discipline, too.

Step 3: Set Clear Goals, and Have a Plan for Execution

In order to continue strengthening your self-discipline, a person must have a clear vision of what goals they are trying to accomplish. They must also have an understanding of what success means to them. If a person doesn't know where they're planning to go or what accomplishing their goals even and Tails, it is easy for them to lose their way or to get sidetracked.

Make sure the goals that you are setting have a clear and concise purpose. For example, don't use goals like, "I want to be rich by the next five years." This goal is too broad for it to have a strong meaning. Instead, you should make a goal that is quantifiable like, "I am planning on saving $20,000 by the end of this year." Then, when you have a quantifiable goal, you are able to make a plan that makes sense for yourself. In this example, a person can plan to save $2,000 each month for the rest of this year in order to hit their goal of saving $20,000 by the end of it. They can break down these goals even further and figure out where in their budget they can save money or how they can make more money to accomplish that goal.

Step 4: Build Your Self-Discipline

Self-discipline is not something that people are born with; it is mostly a learned behavior. Self-discipline is just like any other skill that people may be looking to grow; it requires repetition and lots of daily practice. Like going to the gym, the more you work out your muscles, the bigger and stronger they will become. Changes do not happen overnight, instead to strengthen your muscles and to grow them; it will take at least several weeks for a person to be able to see their progress. The effort and focus that training self-discipline requires can be extremely tiring.

The more time you practice self-discipline, it can become more and more difficult to keep utilizing your willpower. Sometimes, when a person is faced with a big temptation or decision, they may feel that overcoming that large temptation makes it harder for them to overcome other tasks that also require self-discipline. The only way to move past this is to have a good mindset. By having a good mindset, it creates a buffer for how quickly your willpower becomes drained. In addition, like the muscle example we used, by exerting your willpower more often, you will have a higher tolerance and therefore be able to exert it more than if you were just starting out.

Step 5: Create New Habits by Keeping It Simple

To strengthen self-discipline, you need to work on instilling a new habit, which can feel very intimidating at first, especially if you are focusing on the entire goal all at once. To avoid this daunting feeling, keep it very simple. Break your bigger goal into smaller doable ones. Instead of trying to accomplish one huge goal all at once or to change all your habits all at once, focus on doing just one thing consistently and exercise your self-discipline with that one small thing.

For example, if you are somebody that is looking to get into better shape, start by exercising for 10 to 15 minutes per day. Instead of trying to go to the gym for 2 hours every day, which can be very daunting, start with a smaller goal in mind first. By taking baby steps, you can get your mind used to that habit and slowly increase the amount of time that you spend at the gym. Eventually, once you feel like that goal has become a habit, you can then begin to focus on other small goals and keep building up words from there.

Step 6: Eat Healthy and Often

We learned in the earlier chapters that glucose levels play a big role in a person's brainpower, which controls a person's willpower. The sensation of being hungry can cause people to feel angry, annoyed, and irritated. This feeling is real, and everyone has felt it before and often has a huge impact on a person's willpower. Research has found evidence that having low blood sugar weakens a person's ability to make good decisions.

When a person is hungry, their ability to concentrate suffers a lot, and their brain doesn't function as optimally. Therefore, a person's self-control is likely to be weakened when their body is in this state. To prevent this, make sure to be eating small meals constantly to prevent yourself from feeling that annoying hungry feeling that causes people to have a lapse in judgment. Since exercising willpower takes up a lot of energy from a person's brain, make sure to keep fueling it with enough glucose so that the brain can keep functioning at an optimal level.

Step 7: Change Your View Regarding Willpower

We learned in the earlier chapters that a person's point of view or their beliefs could create a buffer of how long it takes to have their willpower drained completely. Although most researchers believe that there is a limit to how much we can tap into our willpower, they also found that the people who believe that there wasn't a limit had a bigger willpower stockpile. If a person believes that they have a limited amount of willpower, they probably will not be able to surpass those limits. However, if a person does not place a strict limit on themselves, they are less likely to use up their willpower stockpile before meeting their goals.

A person's internal perception about their own willpower and self-control plays a huge role in determining how much willpower they have. If a person can remove these obstacles by believing that they have a large stockpile of willpower, then they are less likely to drain out their willpower compared to someone who believes that they don't have much of it. Hence, try changing your own perception of how you see your willpower. Try to think of it as a source that can run out, but because of your beliefs, you have a larger amount of it. This is a much better mindset to be in compared to thinking that willpower will run out, so therefore, you should be stingy with it.

Step 8: Make a Backup Plan

Many psychologists use a famous technique that helps with boosting willpower called "implementation intention." This technique is where you give yourself a plan when you are faced with a potentially difficult situation. We used this example earlier, if a person is trying to reduce the amount of alcohol that they drink and they know that they are going to a party where they will be asked if they want to drink alcohol, instead of always asking for a beer like they normally do, they will instead ask for a plain soda with lime.

By making a plan before going to a situation that you know where you will be confronted with big temptations, you will have an action plan in place where you can automatically use rather than having to come up with an excuse on the spot and risking failure. When a person goes into those situations with a plan, it helps give them the mindset and the self-control that is necessary to overcome obstacles. They will be able to save energy by not having to make sudden decisions or make sudden plans based on their emotional state. This will make them less likely to cave into temptations and more likely to exercise their self-discipline.

Step 9: Reward Yourself

Just like anything else in life, it is necessary to give yourself a break and to give yourself a reward. Give yourself something to look forward to by planning an appropriate reward when you accomplish your goals. This is not much different from when you were a little kid, and you got a treat from your parents for showing good behavior. When a person has something to look forward to, it gives them the extra motivation that they need to succeed.

Anticipation is a powerful thing. It gives people something to focus on so that they are not only thinking of all the things that they need to change. When you have achieved one of your goals, you can find yourself a new goal and a new reward in order to keep motivating yourself to move forward. However, the reward should not be something unhealthy. For example, in the previous example of the person that is trying to lower their alcohol intake, their reward for not drinking as often should not be that they will go binge drinking next Friday. Their awards should be something healthy that won't make them lose progress on all the work that they've done.

Step 10: Forgive Yourself, and Keep Moving Forward

Even if a person has all the best intentions and the most well-made plans, sometimes they will fall short when practicing self-discipline. Avoiding failure altogether is impossible, and we should not build a mindset around that. Everyone will have their ups and downs, their successes, and their failures. The key to overcoming the failures that you will face is just to keep moving forward. If you stumble on your journey of self-discipline, instead of giving up altogether, acknowledge what caused it, learn from it, and then move on. Don't let yourself get caught up in frustration, anger, or guilt because these emotions are the ones that will de-motivate you and get in the way of your future progress. Learn from the mistakes you have made and be comfortable with forgiving yourself. Once you have done that, you can get your head back in the game and start where you left off.

Chapter 5: Tips and Habits to Build Self-Discipline

At this point in the book, you have learned the ten major steps that a person can take to achieve stronger self-discipline. All these steps are pretty basic, and any person, no matter how experienced or inexperienced, would be able to follow them without much difficulty. We are going to take this a little bit further, and I'm going to provide you with a few more tips and habits that will help you to strengthen your self-discipline even more. If you've ever read any psychology books in the past, you would know that a lot of what a person does every day is very habit driven. You might even know, from your own experience, that some people don't like to stray away from their habits and routines. This means that if a person develops the right habits, they would be able to have stronger self-discipline without feeling like they are draining their willpower. People tend to lose self-discipline when they feel like their willpower has been drained, and they can no longer resist the temptations in their lives.

So, where do habits come from, and how are they developed? Why is it that when many people try to change their habits by breaking the bad ones or building good ones that they only stick with it for a certain amount of time before they give up and go back to their old ways? The biggest problem here, especially with habits that people have had for many years or even decades, are the neural pathways that have been imprinted into people's brains. This happens on a biological level. These neural pathways are responsible for linking up the neural networks in a person's brain to perform a specific function like preparing a cup of coffee in a certain way, walking up the stairs, or smoking a cigarette.

These neural pathways help a person automate behavior that is constantly used to reduce the energy needed for the conscious processing power in a person's brain. By doing this, it allows a person's mind to focus on other things rather than the habitual tasks that they have done a thousand times. This function stems from our early days as humans and his part of our DNA; it allows humans to have a more efficient mind that can be used for other things rather than mundane things.

In this case, it's normally the mundane behaviors that are often repeated, which hold people back from building good habits in most cases. People tend to have more bad habits that are adding negative value to their lives rather than good habits that help them achieve their goals further. Since the cause of this is the neural pathways that get ingrained deeper and deeper over time, it makes it harder for people to break their bad habits or even form good ones when all the bad ones are constantly getting in the way. However, if you can try to ingrain the next following habits we will be discussing into your life, you will find that strengthening your self-discipline may become easier. Again, these things don't happen overnight. Remember that habits take lots of time to form and even to break. If you start small and take baby steps and build, you will stop thinking about how much longer you can discipline yourself since you will have ingrained those habits into your brain, which then automatically promotes the self-discipline that you seek.

Habit #1: Gratitude

Gratitude is an important action in human life that helps not only people with self-discipline but is often used to help people that are facing self-esteem and self-confidence issues. A huge problem in our modern world today is that we are constantly presented with millions of materialistic things that cause us always to be wanting something more or something else. This causes people to spend too much time thinking about all the things that they want, and not enough time thinking about the things that they already have. Building a habit of gratitude helps people move away from constantly wanting the things that they don't have and move forward towards appreciating the things that they do have. When people do this, they can begin to make remarkable changes in their lives.

The effects of practicing and showcasing gratitude are extremely crucial. It improves people's mental health, emotional well-being, and spirituality—gratitude is capable of so many things. Practicing gratitude is an exercise that is constantly used in therapy to help the client move away from thinking about things that aren't in the present and focus on being mindful. Most importantly, gratitude helps people move away towards a state of abundance and away from a state of lack. When people live in a state of lack, it makes it impossible for them to focus on achieving their goals and being self-disciplined. They spend too much of their mental energy and capacity worrying about the things that they don't have or living in a fearful way, to the point that they forget about the things that they do have.

The state of lack can also show up in someone as physical symptoms. This state produces a lot of stress because the brain automatically releases cortisol and epinephrine, which are the stress hormones from our brains. These hormones impact numerous systems within the human body. When someone is stressed, their immune systems, digestive systems, and reproductive systems are all affected. We must spend a few minutes every day writing down all the things that we are grateful for. Even if you feel like you don't have anything to be grateful for, try hard to find something. It doesn't have to be anything large, like winning the lottery or finding $20 on the ground. It could be something very simple like the nice weather, the nice conversation that you had with your barista, or even just seeing a cute dog on your way home.

Habit #2: Forgiveness

If you are someone living a fast-paced life, how often do you find yourself feeling angry, frustrated, or annoyed? Due to the insane amount of convenience we are offered in our daily lives, simple annoyances that happen in a person's day can cause a spiral of negative emotions. For example, if you are in a hurry to get to work and you happen to be running late that day, the coffee shop that you normally stop at to get your morning coffee is taking forever to make your order. When you finally get your coffee, you realize that they had made your order wrong, but now, you have no time to get it fixed. That one simple human error has spent you into a spiral of anger and annoyance, and you struggle to let go of it, and you find that it is still negatively impacting your whole day. This causes you to have spent most of your energy upset about the coffee shop that wronged you, and you don't have enough mental capacity to focus on other things like practicing your self-discipline. When people spend most of their days feeling the emotions of anger, regret, or guilt, they are creating more problems than they are with solutions. The emotions of anger and hate consume much more energy in a person's body compared to positive emotions like forgiveness and love. Forgiveness is something that can be learned. When people learn to forgive, only then will they be able to let go of certain things.

Without learning the habit of forgiveness, people would simply not be able to achieve self-discipline. When a person is too worried about how someone or something has wronged them, it makes it impossible for them to focus on achieving their goals or on their personal discipline. If someone has hurt you in the past, learn to forgive them. It doesn't mean that you must forget about what they did to you altogether. Simply just forgive and let go of that negative energy and give it back to the universe rather than keeping it within your body. When we perform the act of forgiveness, we are letting go of the negative energy that inhibits our ability to practice self-discipline. If you want to master self-discipline, you must get rid of sources that are sucking away at your mental energy. Holding on to negative emotions like anger is a sure way for your energy to be drained. While forgiveness might not seem like a discipline habit when you first look at it, it is an extremely crucial one to build in the process.

Try to think about the people or situations that you are currently angry with. It could be someone that you think has wronged you recently, or simply just an annoying situation that has happened to you. Instead of just thinking about how it made you feel, try to put yourself in their shoes. What would be the things that you would do if you were in their situation? Make it light-hearted and try to find some humor in it. Rather than thinking about it as a situation that shouldn't have happened, try to find a lesson learned in those situations. I know that it is very hard to forgive certain people, especially if they have really hurt you or wronged you in life. However, it isn't until people are able to let go of those feelings of animosity and hurt before things in their life really began to improve. People are often so busy stressing and worrying that they don't spend enough time thinking about how they are going to change their future.

Habit #3: Meditation

Just like gratitude, meditation is a commonly used technique to help people practice mindfulness in cases where they are suffering from an anxiety disorder or depression disorder. Meditation is something that can be used to help put people's minds at ease. Provide people with a spiritual centeredness that can be used as an avenue of growth. When people meditate, they take their awareness away from things of the past and the future and focus it on the things of the present. When this happens, they are able to connect themselves to the universe, which also helps them with increasing gratitude.

In the later chapters of this book, we will learn the specific ways of how meditation can help a person improve their self-discipline. Meditation actually plays a big role in a person's ability to use their willpower. Its function is to clear the mind of any thoughts and simply focus all attention on the present. From a self-discipline perspective, meditation helps set the right tone for a person's day. In addition, it helps people improve their physical, emotional, and mental health all at once, allowing them to gain some of the biggest benefits for the least amount of time invested.

There are many types of meditation—some of which focus on mindfulness, and some of which focus on love and gratitude. There truly are too many different types of meditation for humankind to keep track of, but the most popular and beneficial type that is used amongst many therapies and within self-discipline is mindfulness meditation. Contrary to common belief, meditation doesn't have to take a long time. It can be done in 10 to 15 minutes. However, the hardest part of meditation is bringing yourself to do it. A person must be able to keep their mind still and train it to stop wandering all the time. The trick behind mindfulness meditation is not to stop wandering thoughts altogether, but simply to acknowledge these thoughts and reroute yourself back to the present. There are many types of breathing techniques that can be accompanied with meditation to help with achieving mindfulness. We will be diving deeper into these techniques in the meditation chapter.

Some people believe that meditation is about aligning the physical human body with its spiritual body. However, for the purpose of this book, we will stay away from spirituality and focus more on the practical benefit that being mindful can bring.

Habit #4: Active Goal setting

We have mentioned this briefly in the previous chapter, but it is important enough that we will mention it again. We learned in the previous chapter that setting attainable goals is more effective than setting Broad and large goals. By setting smaller goals, it becomes something that is more quantifiable, and because of this, you can easily keep track of how you are doing when it comes to goal achievement.

Active goal setting is very different from passive goal setting. Passive goal setting means you are setting goals in your mind, and they are passive because they lack many details are planning. Passive goal setting means that a person hasn't properly defined the actual goal, which makes it hard for them to keep track of their progress and knowing what needs to be done in order to achieve that goal. Active goal setting is the complete opposite of passive goal setting. Active goal setting means writing out these goals and making sure that they have an important meeting. These goals have to be measurable and very specific. To successfully have an active goal, a person has to make a plan towards achieving it. This is why people set long-term goals, but also engage in smaller goals on a daily basis in order to work towards achieving the bigger goal.

By using active goal setting, it ingrains the discipline in us because you are forced to give it direction. By breaking down your big goals into smaller daily goals, it helps people avoid distractions by only looking at the things that they need to get done in the present day. This way, a person isn't left constantly thinking about one large intimidating goal but not knowing how to approach it.

Active goal setting works by taking the first step in setting your long-term goals. If you are someone that has long-term goals like; wanting to own your first home, wanting to pay off your student debt by the next three years, or wanting to take 6 months off to travel Europe. If you are someone that has long-term goals, then you need to actively participate in daily, weekly, and monthly goal setting and planning. You have to play an active role in tracking your progress towards your goals and making changes in places wherein you feel like things aren't working for you.

So, take out a pen and a piece of paper and start writing down what long-term goals you have. Once you have some long-term goals written down, break it down into monthly, weekly, and daily goals. Start slowly by accomplishing your daily goals, and when you reach the end of the month, assess to see if you have achieved your monthly goal through accomplishing your daily goals. If you haven't, look back on your daily goals and see if there's anything you can change so that you could achieve next month's goal.

Habit #5: Eating Healthy

We also discussed the benefits of eating healthy in the previous chapter, but we will expand on it a little bit more here. What a lot of people don't realize is that our human body spends a huge portion of its energy digesting and processing food. When a person's diet is rich in proteins, fats, and carbohydrates, their body is actually using more energy to process food—some of which is useless to us.

Raw fruits and foods actually offer the biggest boost of energy for humans because they require less energy for the body to process and provides more energy for the body to use after that. This process is called an enhanced Thermic Effect of Food (TEF) or otherwise known as Dietary Induced Thermogenesis (DIT).

Like we learned in the previous chapter, our brains use up a large amount of glucose in order to keep it functioning. Therefore, the amount of energy that a person has is very responsible and how focused they feel. When a person is focused, they can achieve their goals using less willpower than if they weren't focused. When a person is feeling too comatose from the unhealthy food that they have eaten, staying focused is something that is very hard to achieve. They often spend too much of their time feeling too sluggish and exhausted to work on achieving their goals.

You commonly hear that breakfast is the most important meal of the day. However, it's important not only to eat a healthy breakfast but to eat multiple healthy meals throughout the day. In order to do this, you have to actively plan what you're going to eat during these meals in order to break some of your bad habits. For example, if you are planning to eat five healthy smaller-sized meals per day, but you haven't prepared any of those meals, you are more likely to feel hungry and indulge in unhealthy conveniences like fast food. If you are someone that eats fast food or processed foods often, your body won't be able to create enough energy to help you approach your goals with focus or help you have the willpower in order to start working at them.

Since the food that a person eats can change the neural chemical makeup of their brain, it also heavily influences a person's mind and body connection. Take a look at the things that you eat during your day. Try to find the meals where you often indulge in unhealthy food or junk food. Plan in advance so you can substitute those meals with raw, organic, and healthy foods. By buying this type of healthy food in advance and preparing it for the times that you become hungry, you will be less likely to visit your nearest McDonalds.

Habit #6: Sleeping

Since the theory behind willpower is that it gets its energy from the brain, which gets its energy from glucose levels and rest, then it's safe to assume that sleep is directly connected to how the brain is able to acquire energy. When a person doesn't get enough sleep, their brain spends most of its energy focused on just keeping your basic body functions up and going. This does not leave much energy for a person to spend on exerting their willpower, practicing self-discipline, or even simply just remembering their self-discipline. Getting the proper and healthy amount of sleep is a vital requirement for accomplishing anything. When a person doesn't get enough sleep, it affects their ability to focus, their judgment, their mood, their overall health, and their diet.

When people suffer chronic sleep deprivation, such as insomnia, things go from bad to worse. Many research studies have found evidence that people who don't get the proper amount of sleep on a regular basis have a greater risk of catching specific diseases. Lack of sleep also has a significant and negative impact on a person's immune system. This can cause a person to frequently catch a common cold or flu, which causes them not to have the ability to go to school, work, or get anything effective done.

For an adult, it is important to get at least six hours of sleep every night. A healthy amount of sleep should range between eight to ten hours every night, but the minimum amount is 6 hours. Avoid eating or drinking anything that contains caffeine at least 5 hours before your bedtime so that it doesn't affect your natural sleep cycle. Make a note to also stay away from ingesting too many toxins during the day such as cigarettes, alcohol, drugs, or prescription medicine if it can be avoided.

In conclusion, the benefits of getting enough sleep are extraordinary. Aside from the fact that it can help you stay focused and be more disciplined, it also helps you to curb inflammation and pain, to lower stress, to improve your memory, to jumpstart your creativity, to sharpen your attention, to improve your grades, to limit your chances for accidents, and to avoid depression.

Habit #7: Exercise

Exercise is one of the most important habits to build within all people. It acts as a cornerstone habit to help a person's life be filled with positive habits and be rid of the bad ones. A person that is truly able to discipline themselves has to instill the habit of exercise into their everyday routine. As you all may already know, there are endless benefits when it comes to exercise. This is something that is talked about not only by psychologists but medical experts as well. Even though exercise is such an important component of a person's life, not everyone actually makes it a priority. Why is this?

In our busy modern-day lives, everyone is caught up with trying to get all the things that they need to get done and are often busy running around completing errands and fail just to tackle exercise head-on. Often, people have a bad mindset when it comes to exercise and think that they won't be able to build it as a habit because they simply have "too many other things to do." This is where most people are wrong. There are ways to incorporate exercise even if their day is jam-packed from beginning to end.

When people think of exercise, they may automatically think of a minimum one-hour intense weight-lifting session at the gym, a one-hour-long, expensive spin class, or a one-hour yoga class. If that's what they are thinking about then yes, it is true that the people that have busy lives may not be able to incorporate the time to get to their exercise class, the time it takes to complete the exercise class, and then get to wherever they need to go after that. However, exercise doesn't necessarily have to be a formalized session that takes a long time. It can simply be getting some sit-ups, push-ups, or some jumping jacks in the morning before you head to work. It can also be you choosing to walk to work instead of taking the bus, or it could be a brief walk around your neighborhood park after dinner.

By instilling exercise as a keystone habit of your life, it can help you become more disciplined and can also improve your life in numerous ways. First of all, exercise is extremely effective in reducing stress levels and pain because it causes the brain to release feel-good endorphins and neurotransmitters like serotonin and dopamine. Secondly, exercise helps increase the oxygenation and blood flow of body cells, which is responsible for helping boost the immune system and fighting off diseases. Lastly, exercise increases a person's ability to focus on the task at hand due to the increased activity in the brain, which allows us to live a more disciplined life.

So start building the habit of exercise in your life by simply just going for a 10-minute walk or just doing some sit-ups and push-ups right after you wake up. Just a few minutes is fine.

Try to do this for one week and then increase the amount of time you spend on that session for the next week. Keep up with this pattern, and soon enough, you will have a healthy amount of time every day that you set aside to get your exercise in, and this is when it will become a full-blown habit.

Habit #8: Organization

Have you ever noticed that when your home is messy, it makes it very hard to be comfortable and therefore leads you to be unfocused and distracted? Naturally, humans don't like living in a dirty and messy environment. In order for a person to achieve their goals and accomplish self-discipline, they need to be organized. Organizing also needs to become a habit that is fully incorporated into a person's personal life and professional life. This includes the physical act of organizing the things you have in your home and the mental act of organizing the things on your mind.

By living an organized life, you are living a disciplined life. If you are constantly scattered and disorganized, start small with your organization skills. Just pick one small space each day for yourself to organize. This can be just one single drawer in your kitchen, the things lying around on your desk, or just straighten out the things on your coffee table. The next day, pick something else to organize like your bathroom drawers or the clothes in your closet. The more time you spend living in a clean and organized environment, the less you would want your home to become cluttered and messy again. You will start to notice when clutter builds up, and by having a habit of organization, you will immediately organize things as you use them so that you don't have to spend time organizing it later on.

By decluttering your home or your working environment, you will have plenty of different areas where you can sit down and work on your own goals. Has your home ever been so cluttered that when you do have the motivation to start working on something, you simply just don't have the space to do it? In order to avoid this, always keep your home clean and organized so that when you have a rush of motivation, you can find a workspace that is clean and ready for you to work.

Like a lot of other habits, the habit of organizing can be learned and built over time. It does require your attention and effort, but it is something that will pay off tremendously in the long run. When you are living in a physical space that is organized and clean, your mind will automatically become more stress-free, relaxed, and give you the ability to focus. In turn, by becoming more organized, you are increasing your ability to be more self-disciplined. Begin to incorporate this good habit of putting things back where it belongs when you're finished using it rather than leaving it out. Little things like this we do daily have the largest impact on the quality of life. Pay attention to small things, and you'll begin to see big benefits.

Habit #9: Time Management

In the busy world that we live in today, time management is extremely crucial if you are trying to get everything that you need to get done. An average person has to work 40 hours a week, not including the time it takes for them to commute to work, and still have to make time for things like exercise, relationships, socializing, family, and achieving the goals that they have set. Without good time management, it will be virtually impossible for anyone to get anything done unless they are able to manage their time effectively.

When people can manage their time properly, they will begin to have room to do the things that actually matter. Mainly, they must make room to do the activities that they need in order to achieve the goals that they have set. For a person to achieve their long-term goals, they have to break it down into smaller daily goals that may not be the most urgent but are definitely still very important. If a person does not have good time management, they likely cannot even get the most urgent things that they need to get done in a day, let alone achieving goals that don't require immediate urgency.

To effectively measure if certain things are urgent, non-urgent, important, not important, you need to take a second to think about whether or not the action that you are doing is not 'urgent but important' or 'not urgent and not important' or 'urgent and important.' The things that fall into the 'not urgent and not important' category are known as things that are time-wasters. This includes things like browsing social media on your phone or binge-watching your favorite Netflix series. Things that fall into the category of 'not urgent but important' are likely the short-term goals you have set for yourself. Although they don't need to be urgently completed, they are still important for your self-growth. Things that are urgent and important are likely deadlines or any responsibilities that you have to complete for your work.

A person's ability to strengthen self-discipline is derived from their ability to manage their time. Some of the most successful people in the world are incredible time managers because, rather than using time as a detractor, they use time as a benefit. Everybody has the same amount of time in a day—we shouldn't waste it. Start managing your time by categorizing the things you need to do in a day with the categories I gave you above. Start by doing the things that are both urgent and important, then move on to the things that are non-urgent but important. Leave the things that are both not urgent or important to the end of the day when you have completed all the other things. This way, you are maximizing your time to get the things that you need to get completed.

Habit #10: Persistence

This last habit you probably saw coming. No amount of self-discipline would ever be complete without the presence of persistence. Persistence is a type of habit that helps us not to give up even when we are faced with failure. Persistence is what helps us get back up on our feet to keep trying even when we do fail. Persistence plays such a huge role in self-discipline that without it, achieving self-discipline is probably impossible.

You might be wondering why that is. This is because achieving our goals is not an easy thing to do. It is really hard. Getting discouraged is easy and something that happens to everyone along their journey. In addition, giving up takes far less energy and effort compared to continuing to push through even if it's something that causes a lot of pain in the process before it can give us any pleasure.

However, this hardship that is required to achieve any goals is simply something that you have to persevere through because that's just what it takes. We all have to realize that even the most successful people in the world have failed numerous times over and over again. Failure is simply a part of life, and rather than avoiding it and not pursuing your goals at all in fear of failure, we should learn to persevere and push through even during the hardest of times. Without fail, we wouldn't be able to achieve the big goals that we have set for ourselves.

There are many ways that a person can go about instilling perseverance as a habit, but the best and most effective weight is to come up with the reasons why you want to do the things in life that you aim for. If the reasons behind your goals are strong enough, they can motivate you so that you can get through anything.

Chapter 6: The Challenges of Self-Discipline

In this chapter, we will focus on learning some of the challenges that come with strengthening your self-discipline. We already know that hardship and failure are a part of the process of life and the process of building self-discipline. By understanding what these challenges might be in advance, it gives you an idea of what to prepare for when you are faced with an obstacle. Like we mentioned earlier in this book, having a plan prepared when you are in the face of a challenge or temptation can help you react in a way that is good rather than in a way that negatively affects your progress.

One problem that people normally face when they are trying to strengthen their self-discipline is falling into a self-defeating loop. It looks like this: fail to engage in the desired behavior → negative physical/psychological consequences → low mood, shame, and self-criticism → low motivation to engage in healthy behaviors. In this chapter, I will be addressing a few challenges that are most commonly experienced when a person is looking to practice their self-discipline.

Fighting Against 'Natural' Tendencies

Oftentimes, people feel like their natural state should be to sit on their couch, with a plethora of snacks, and watching their favorite TV show. During those days, the idea of going to the gym or even just eating a healthy meal seems to be totally absurd. It is interesting that people nowadays have been conditioned by the expectations of society to think that their natural state is lazy. We live in a world where if you are not constantly on-the-go or working your butt off at work, then you are not working hard enough. The result of these feelings is that people tend to get trapped, thinking that practicing self-discipline is the constant battle of fighting against a person's natural state. Their mindset is one that is a psychological battle of laziness versus self-discipline. Having this type of mindset makes it difficult to practice self-discipline.

One of the reasons that I suspect behind this mindset is the fact that people tend to mistake the need for rest to laziness. Lots of mental or physical exertion creates fatigue in the human body. Rest is a recovery process so that the person can not only get stronger but also be able to repeat and exceed that mental and physical exertion. If your mindset regarding self-discipline is one that is constant and uninterrupted work, then you deny your body's natural need for recovery and rest. This need for recovery will show itself as a type of sabotage of your self-discipline efforts, and you will automatically label it as being lazy. Be careful when this happens, as this label is very incorrect.

Rather than mistaking any urges of rest as a sign of being lazy, think about whether or not you have exerted yourself already. If so, it is all right to stop what you're doing and take a quick break to recharge. Getting into the mindset that you are lazy, or that resting is for lazy people, then you will always feel negative about yourself every time your body shows you a natural symptom when it is asking you to rest.

The World Doesn't Care About Your Attempts at Self-Discipline

When a person makes a decision to actively and purposefully restructure their life and behavior, the universe doesn't just magically make things easier for them. On the contrary, it will likely throw many challenges at you. It may rain the day that you decide to go out for a run, or your coworker might buy you a whole box of chocolates just to be nice on the day that you decide to eat healthily.

Since the world isn't built on fairness or justice or reward, it is silly to think that the universe will consciously support the changes that you are trying to make in your life. There are people who claim that the universe is presenting opportunities to them when they have decided to change their life. This is inaccurate because if a person is looking to change their life, they likely have taken on new activities. By being exposed to new people and new information, this is what creates new opportunities that have nothing to do with the universe trying to help you. So, don't spend time thinking about whether or not your self-discipline plan is something that the universe will help you with. Instead, spend your time preparing for all the obstacles that will get in your way of achieving your goals. If you do run into obstacles, which you will, don't think that they were placed there deliberately to throw you off, but they were already there in the first place.

Difficulty Breaking Well-Worn Emotional Behavior Pathways

One of the most well-known concepts in Psychology is that the emotions that people feel are very powerful influences on their behavior. These emotions and feelings are developed over the course of human evolution in order to help us with survival. Negative emotions that people often feel like fear and anxiety lets them know that danger is nearby. Feelings of happiness or excitement tell us that it's okay to approach the situation. The feeling of anger lets us know that it may be an opportunity where we would need to fight. Sadness lets us know when we need to seek comfort from our loved ones.

However, as people, we have learned that emotions and feelings aren't always the best guide to how we behave. People may get anxious in situations that don't actually have any real danger, or they may get angry in situations where fighting isn't an appropriate reaction. Over the course of our lives, we've learned to pick up different habits of ways to react when it comes to responding and managing our emotions. For example, if someone had a rough day after work, their habitual behavior would be to drink a couple of glasses of wine. They do this because this action has worked for them in the past, but they may not realize that they need to change it when they may have outgrown his habit. Some people may try to numb their feelings of sadness or stress by scrolling on their phones in order to prevent themselves from thinking about other things.

Oftentimes, these types of emotional habits derived from the roots of somebody's childhood, where they first learned how to deal with their emotions. Without knowing, people may learn that numbing their emotions is the best strategy for not dealing with the negative ones, or they may try to distract themselves with unhealthy things like alcohol or food. These strategies become reinforced when a person repeatedly uses them and has received success in the past from it. By the time children become adults, they have built some emotion to behavior pathways that are not very well-established and hard to break. This is why people have so much trouble when it comes to strengthening their self-discipline because habits that have formed over the decades require lots of time and willpower to break down and be rebuilt.

In the process of establishing new habits, it also means that people will have to confront their well-worn habit. For example, if a person's goal was to eat healthily and get in shape, they may have to face their habit of comforting themselves with food and abandon it altogether. Although it may not seem like this is an emotional event, people subconsciously grow very attached to their coping mechanisms. By giving that up altogether, people often feel like they are stripped of their safety net. This means that strengthening and practicing self-discipline is very hard and emotional work. The emotions and feelings that people have managed through using their own coping mechanisms now become very apparent to them because the coping mechanism has been removed. This typically doesn't make people very happy, and they often have trouble dealing with their emotions without the safety net that they would always fall back on.

By understanding this important concept, you can prepare yourself for the difficulties that you will face when you are practicing your self-discipline. Some of the practices and work that you put in will be very emotionally challenging. You may be able to initiate changes in your life using some simple and concrete goals that you've made for yourself, but you may quickly learn that if there is emotional baggage, you would have to face them head-on along your journey.

Being Self-Disciplined Does Not Make You a Popular Person

When people first begin practicing self-discipline and are excited to make him good changes in their lives, they often hope that their efforts will inspire other people to get into good habits as well. They think that by changing into a better person and achieving the goals that they've always wanted to achieve for themselves and that they will gain respect from other people. This thought process is normal because why wouldn't you want to share with your loved ones that you are changing your life for the better?

However, in reality, most people will just think that the person who is trying to change is annoying because they go from being easy-going about what they eat to having major food restrictions if they are trying to change their diet. They will begin saying no to certain activities that get in the way of them achieving their goals. They will begin to prioritize other important things regarding the goals that they are going after rather than spending time with people that may not be exactly beneficial to them. Being self-disciplined is not something that is going to make a person more likable.

In order to be a socially desirable person, you have to be willing to spend a lot of your time with other people doing things that are often unhealthy, like eating out and drinking socially. Let's say that this person manages to strike a really good balance between achieving their goals and still remaining socially desirable. Any success that they achieve isn't necessarily going to inspire others. This is because of two reasons. The first reason is that people won't really care because most of the time they have their own problems to deal with. The second reason is that watching someone else have success when it comes to achieving goals while they're struggling with their own goals is not always inspirational; they may even see it as annoying. People may even consciously or unconsciously attempt to throw you off track because they can't bear to look at their own lives due to jealousy or other emotions.

Just to clarify, other people may not be trying to throw you off track maliciously. I don't think that people would intentionally want you to fail. However, I do think that your attempts at practicing self-discipline to take control of your own life is not something that gets you admiration and respect from other people. Relationships are very complex interactions. The message I'm trying to get across here is that self-discipline should be something that you pursue for yourself and for your own intrinsic reasons. You should not be doing it to seek congratulation or respect from others because you will likely get the opposite.

Motivation and Inspiration May Be Totally Absent

Some people may have multiple goals that they are looking to achieve. For example, it could be a mix of getting more exercise, eating healthier, pursuing a musical instrument, and being successful in their career. However, it may be that not all those things can create inspiration or motivation. Out of those goals, there may only be one item that produces the most inspiration and motivation for a person.

Somewhere along the way of self-discipline, a lot of people realize that motivation and inspiration actually precede action. With this belief comes the expectation that the presence of inspiration and motivation will tell people what they need to do with their lives. They think that wherever there are motivation and inspiration, that is the direction that they should be heading. Although this is a lovely notion, it is not one that lines up with reality. Take someone's university degree as an example. I can almost guarantee that there were many days where a person doesn't feel inspired or motivated to do their schoolwork, but it doesn't change the reality that having a university degree is a very beneficial addition to your life. If a person were to be using motivation and inspiration as a guide, that degree likely wouldn't be finished.

A person's choices of where they focus their self-discipline do need to be carefully selected and initiated using the most logical thinking that they can muster. People may try to eat healthily or work out frequently in order to have a healthy body, but that does not mean that they are inspired to do it. Keep in mind that I am not saying that inspiration and motivation are worthless feelings. What I am trying to get across here is that the presence of these two feelings can be an unreliable source for somebody to make decisions regarding their life. For some people, inspiration and motivation don't show up until they have already put in quite a bit of work towards their goals. For example, somebody who is looking to get more muscular might not actually feel motivated to work out until they got into a regular habit of lifting weights at the gym.

You Might Not Be Doing the Right Things

If you have tried to achieve a goal using various different types of angles, but you are constantly failing repeatedly at a certain area of self-discipline, you might have to face the possibility that you have selected something that you simply might not ever be able to engage in on a regular basis. Self-discipline is not only about picking a goal or an activity and doing it despite all costs. Self-discipline is about picking the important activities and goals and doing them against all obstacles. It may be a possibility that you have simply picked a goal or activity that isn't all that important to you. It is all right to admit that and move forward. The good thing about this is that if it turns out the goal our activity was important to you, after all, it will pop up in your life again thematically, and you would be able to take it up again.

Self-Discipline Fatigue

As we have learned in the earlier chapters of this book, it is extremely tiring and exhausting to be consciously fighting temptation and selecting healthy activities and choosing the productive activities over the unproductive ones. It is tiring because it constantly drains on your willpower resources. It takes lots of energy and effort to turn away from the wrong choices and pick the ones that are right for your goals. It takes lots of resistance to choose healthy food over unhealthy food that may be quicker and much more convenient. It takes a lot of effort to drag yourself out of bed on a rainy morning to get to the gym to work out rather than sleeping an extra hour.

The only way to really battle this problem is to practice your required tasks until they become a habit. You want those daily tasks that you need to do to reach a level of automation that you no longer actively think about it, and it no longer consumes your willpower resources. Some people may think that all they need is a few weeks or even just a few months to build a new habit. This mindset is absolutely wrong. The reason why our bad habits are so hard to break is that they have been built up through multiple years. Good habits will take the exact same amount of time. If you have been repeatedly binge-eating whenever you feel upset for the last 10 years of your life, except that it will take multiple years before you can break out of that habit and into a healthy eating habit. However, once you do get into that stage, you no longer have to make decisions about that have it anymore, and they will function on its own.

The good thing is that eventually, with repeated practice, and some failures and obstacles along the way, new and better behaviors will become a habit. When this happens, it will consume far less mental resources than it did before. For instance, you probably don't feel stressed out or tired by the idea that you have to brush your teeth at least twice a day. However, if someone asked you to simply workout for 10 minutes a day, which is the same amount of time that brushing your teeth takes, you may find this much harder to do because it isn't already a habit. Like I mentioned before, it just takes a significant amount of time before a new behavior becomes a learned behavior.

Here are some ways that you can address the fatigue that self-discipline may bring:

- There are days where you should incorporate into your schedule where you can relax and don't have to worry about the things that you have to do in order to reach your goals like dieting or exercising. You can call these 'cheat days' or 'treat days.'

- You can incorporate something called the 80% rule. This means that you are accepting that you won't be a perfect 100% all the time with your tasks or goals and getting 80% on your goals is acceptable.

- Make sure that you were getting enough rest and sleep. We learned that this is your body's and mind's time to recover from the fatigue that we have put it through daily.

Overall, self-discipline is a very important and beneficial thing that you should be incorporating in your life. I truly believe that anything and amazing in life requires a lot of practice and focus. Having the ability to focus on the things that are most important to us and being able to do them on a regular basis even when we are approached with numerous problems and obstacles are the fundamental components of self-worth and self-esteem. Please keep in mind that this process is not going to be an easy one. There are always going to be many failures along your journey, and people often experience failures on a weekly or monthly basis. You should make it a goal to openly accepting and acknowledging some of the difficulties that you have faced along the way to achieving your goals. Just know that you are not alone, and people have likely faced the exact same problems that you are facing now.

Chapter 7: How to Use Visualization to Achieve Your Goals

Most people have tried to visualize their goals at least a couple of times in their lives. They probably spend a lot of time visualizing a desired future event. For the general public, visualization is a process where they picture their future within their minds. However, visualization can be used for so many more things. Visualization is a type of inner transformation that leads to the realization of external results. It's also known as a form of creative thinking or consciously making and shaping your life with a purpose in mind. The best part about the image that a person may have envisioned is that it doesn't have to rely upon the external events of reality. It can be entirely dependent on the imaginative powers of a person.

Within a person's inner world, they can be anyone or anything that they decide to be. It doesn't matter what is happening externally, as it doesn't make a difference to the conscious process of visualization. You might be thinking that this sounds very airy-fairy. However, don't get confused here; visualization is not just a fantasy that someone made up. It is a proactive and very conscious activity where a person can actively visualize things or events in their mind in a specific way to help them impact their external reality positively. Therefore, there is a strong connection between visualization and the real world that we live in, but it does not have to depend on that world entirely. Visualization argues that how a person behaves within the outer world of reality is dependent on how the person creates their internal world for themselves every day.

The Key to Improved Performance Is Visualization

Here is something that I bet not many people know: Visualizing an action or a skill before actually performing that action is just as powerful as doing that action in real life. Scientific research has found tons of evidence that people's thoughts create the exact same instructions in their mind as it does with actions. This means that when somebody is rehearsing or practicing an action in their mind using visualization, it impacts the many cognitive processes within a person's brain that includes planning, motor control, memory, and attention perception. In layman's terms, a person's brain is activated in the exact same manner when they are visualizing an action compared to when they are doing that action physically. Ultimately, scientists can safely assume that the act of visualization is just as valuable as physically performing an action.

Many athletes in certain sports use the act of visualization to help themselves train before a competition. For example, in Olympic cycling, the cyclist will prepare for a competition by closing their eyes and visualizing the racetrack in their mind. They move their bodies while visualizing the way that they will travel through the racetrack in order to train their muscle memory and reflexes even further. This way, when they do begin to compete on the racetrack, they have already visualized themselves cycling through it using the strategies that they have been taught and visualized in their minds. This is a technique and training skill that many professional coaches teach their athletes to do.

When a person is visualizing, their conscious mind is actively aware that the things they're visualizing is not real but is just produced via imagination. Despite this, a person's subconscious doesn't have the ability to identify the difference between what a person is imagining and what they are doing. In other words, a person's inner mind isn't able to distinguish the difference between real life, an imagined future, or a past memory. Rather, the mind is under the impression that everything a person sees is real. This is proven by numerous brain scans that scientists have conducted over the years, where they discovered that there is no difference in brain activity when someone is observing something in the real world compared to when a person is visualizing.

All of this evidence is extremely important because it points the theory that by using visualization, people can develop skills that are completely new to them and be able to reprogram and rewire their mind without the requirement of performing those actions physically. For example, if somebody is looking to increase their self-esteem, then they start by boosting their self-esteem using the process of visualization by imagining themselves doing those actions before doing it in the real world.

Just like how this method is effective for a person to increase their self-esteem, this is also very helpful for people that are looking to increase their self-discipline because it helps minimize the feelings of anxiety. By using the technique of working through scenarios in a person's mind can help them effectively require their brain in order to build new patterns, habits, and behaviors, which makes completing tasks in the real world far less anxiety ridden. Due to this, you will feel much calmer when you bring those performances into your real life.

How Worries Are Reprogramming Your Brain

When a person is experiencing negative emotions like anxiety, fear, worry, or stress, it is a form of negative visualization. It is an unconscious type of visualization where a person is not aware that they are negatively visualizing, but it is still a type of visualizing, nonetheless. Every time a person stresses or worries about something, they often suffer from having anxiety or fear about what they think the future holds, they are in a moment of negative visualization. In addition, at that moment, the person is rewiring their own brain in limiting ways. It is exactly like how a person's mind can be reprogrammed to foster positive habits; it is also able to be reprogrammed negatively.

When a person indulged in the negative worries that they're feeling in the moment, they are building on the existing neural pathways within their brain. Due to this, every time a person envisions something negative, it makes it easier for them to have the same future worries. A person's negative visualizations can make a person feel uneasy or anxious at that moment. The thing that makes it worse is that a person's subconscious doesn't have the ability to tell the difference between a visualization and what the person sees. Due to this, the person's brain views those events as if it is happening in real life, which causes the neural networks to be formed in their brain, which creates new beliefs, habits of behaviors, and perspectives. In plain English, the person is effectively building new patterns by rewiring their brain to support all the things that they have negatively envisioned.

When a person does that, it means they are developing a behavior or skill that is unhelpful. The more often that this person thinks about this pattern, the easier it is for their mind to keep replaying that pattern repeatedly until the action of worrying becomes a habit that is triggered when a person faces any level of uncertainty. In addition to this, when a person worries about certain things, those specific things have a higher chance of manifesting in their daily life. This is due to a person's Reticular Activating System, which happens when a person begins to focus on negative things. Their brain is now searching for anything possible within a person's reach that would support those worries. Due to this, everything a person sees will then validate all the things that they worry about. In addition, every time a person makes bad decisions or choices based on their flawed perspective, it leads to them have their worries manifested into their real world.

This all sounds very incredible, I know. The best part about this is that the exact process that is at play when someone is visualizing negative things also works in a positive way with the goals that they want to achieve. This process initiates the Reticular Activating System, which helps people become more aware of the events, opportunities, and other people that are related to their goals. This leads to the person making conscious and subconscious choices based on that information, which helps them achieve their goals. Due to this, visualization is often accidentally used in a negative way, but it can also be used in a very helpful and empowering way. Whichever one you choose is a choice you can make.

Positive Visualization Techniques

In this chapter, we will be looking at four different types of visualization techniques that a person can use to help improve their life. These techniques include:

- Mastering a new skill

- Healing your mind and body

- Achieving your goals

- Creating a plan

We will be learning about the process of the steps that a person can follow in each of those areas while also discussing the benefits of those techniques. Let's dive right in.

Mastering a New Skill

One way a person can learn a new skill is to utilize visualization. The technique of visualization is extremely effective when a person is learning new skills. This is because the way the brain is activated is just the same as when someone is visualizing the skill and when they physically do that skill. For instance, a study that an Australian psychologist did that studied the visualization technique in regard to a person's ability to accomplish free throws in basketball. This is when a player in a basketball team shoots the ball from the free-throw line after the referee calls a foul during a game.

This psychologist chose three groups of students at random who have never tried visualization before. The first group practiced the skill of free throwing for 3 weeks straight. The second group only practiced free throws twice, once on the first day and once on the last day. The third group did the same. However, the people in the third group visualized free throw for thirty minutes every single day. If they had "missed" in their visualized free throw, they "practiced" getting the free throw right the next shot. On the last day of this experiment, the psychologist measured how the participants improved using percentages. The group that got physical practice every day improved their free throws by 24%. The second group that only practiced twice did not improve at all. However, the third group that had practiced just as much as the second group did perform better by 23%, which is almost as good as the first group. At the end of this experiment, the psychologist published a paper that was about how most effective visualization happens when the visualizer can see what they are doing. In other words, the ones that practiced visualizing the free-throw actually 'felt' the basketball in their hands and 'saw' it going through the hoop and heard it 'bouncing.'

You can also use visualization to learn and master any skill of your liking. The most important thing is to try to utilize all your senses when you begin your visualization. Here are five simple steps to teach you how to visualize properly:

1. Pick a skill that is of interest to you.

2. Identify what your real-world proficiency level is in this skill.

3. Visualize yourself doing this skill using all five of your senses in as much detail as possible.

4. Perform this visualization for 11 days at 20 minutes per day.

5. Try this skill in reality and keep track of measuring your improvement. Continue visualizing while doing that skill in real life if you are not satisfied with the results.

Creating A Plan

Whenever you are feeling stressed and/or overwhelmed, visualization can be a great way to help you build a plan that helps you take proactive action and to stay centered. This visualization technique is most effective when practiced at the end of the day, so you can use it to begin planning the work for your next day. You don't have to be too strict with this as you can also choose to use this technique throughout your day whenever you have a few minutes of free time.

Below are three simple steps to do this:

1. Calm yourself down, and make sure you are feeling relaxed. Sit down as it will help you get some rest from whatever you were doing before.

2. Close your eyes and start to visualize, specifically the things that you are looking to accomplish for the rest of your day and tomorrow. Visualize every action that you need to take in specific detail and then ask yourself the following questions:

    a. How do I want to feel?

    b. What do I want?

    c. How will I interact with others?

    d. What specific actions do I want to take?

    e. How will I overcome obstacles?

    f. What obstacles will I potentially face?

    g. What do I want to achieve?

3. The reality here is that people are not able to predict all the things that might happen to them. When events happen unexpectedly, they can often ruin any plans that have been put in place. However, good planning isn't about planning around all possible obstacles, but it is more about adapting to the obstacles that life gives you. When you keep this in mind, it is important that you affirm with yourself at the end of your visualization

with "this or something better will come my way." By giving yourself affirmation, you are maintaining an open mind for the endless possibilities to come. This will help you feel more prepared and comfortable with making changes when unexpected things happen to you.

This process is definitely not a foolproof plan. However, this visualization will help you to envision possible situations that might happen.

Achieving Your Goals

This visualization technique is the most important one when it comes to strengthening self-discipline. By using the technique of visualization for setting goals brings a lot of value, but this technique does come with one major drawback. The most popular form of visualization is goal-setting. Most people have used visualization pertaining to their goals at one time or another. However, this technique may not have worked for them due to one critical flaw. This flaw is that when people are visualizing their goals, they often are only visualizing their goals at the end. They imagine their flashy goal at the end of all the hard work that's going to be rainbows and butterflies. Yes, they are experiencing this using all their sensory glands, but they simply open their eyes after the visualization feeling very inspired. However, this type of motivation is extremely short-lived because the next time this person faces an obstacle, it immediately deflates their motivation.

When this happens, people need to visualize their goals all over again in order to create more motivation for themselves. However, because nothing happens after every visualization, their motivation stays stagnant and does not grow, and therefore, their hunger towards achieving that goal is not growing as well. In fact, every time a person hits an obstacle and they try the process of visualization again, their motivation becomes weaker every time, and as time goes on, they begin to lose energy as well. So what are they doing incorrectly?

What they are incorrectly doing is that they are not visualizing their goals properly. They only see the destination, but they don't understand that achieving a goal requires much more than just that. The journey of achieving a goal is full of wins and losses, highs and lows, and a journey that is jam-packed with ups and downs. Due to this, these are the things that a person would also need to include in their visualization.

When a person visualizes their end goal, it is very effective in creating that desire and hunger. However, the proper way to use visualization is to spend just 10 percent of your time visualizing the end goal and spending the leftover 90% of the time visualizing the 'how' behind achieving your goals. This will include visualizing yourself, overcoming challenges, and facing setbacks and problems. In some ways, it's like the form of visualization planning that we just discussed.

A person's end goal creates the inspiration that they need long-term, but the actual journey itself helps a person stay motivated in the short term. If you are trying to maximize the time that you spend on achieving small goals to get to your end goal, you must visualize those as well.

Below are five steps that you can follow to achieve this visualization:

1. Get yourself to a quiet place and sit down and shut your eyes. Start to imagine what your end goal will look like. Imagine yourself experiencing and living this goal using all five of your senses.

2. Slowly begin to take steps back from your end goal and imagine the process that you took in order to achieve your end goal. Imagine yourself overcoming all the problems and obstacles that you had to face. Keep visualizing every single step until you find yourself back into your present moment.

3. Move forward in time now and visualize how you took advantage of opportunities and the happy coincidences that aided you in overcoming any barriers. Try to see as clearly as possible how things unfolded for you.

4. At the end of your visualization, take a few moments to send your future self some positive energy for their journey.

5. When you exit the visualization, immediately detach yourself emotionally from the outcome of your goal. One thing that can hold you back is if you are having an emotional attachment to a specific result. Instead, try to stay open-minded and be flexible for the journey ahead.

You can use visualization using those steps on a daily or weekly basis. Your weekly sessions can be as long as 30 minutes, and you can keep your daily sessions shorter so that they are between 5–10 minutes. However, be sure that you are focusing your daily sessions on achieving the next steps of your goal for that specific day or upcoming week. This will keep you moving forward towards your goal. Then, you can focus your weekly visualizations using the five steps above.

Healing Your Mind and Body

Over the last few years of science and research, scientists have found that there is an incredibly strong connection between the human body and the human mind. In fact, this connection is proven to do too many scientific experiments where placebos were used in place of actual medication. In these experiments, the people who took the placebo, believing that they were taking medication, felt improvement. The most interesting part of these experiments is that it has proved that placebos work just as well as the actual medication itself. So what exactly is happening here?

Essentially what is happening behind this healing method is that people are able to convince themselves when something is supposed to help them. As a result, their brain releases the necessary chemicals and neurotransmitters that begin the healing process. There is also an effect called the nocebo effect; this is when a person receives a sugar pill, thinking that it is an actual medication, and as a result of it, they end up feeling worse than before and experiencing the supposed symptoms of this drug. Just like a placebo, a person's brain and their belief systems are responsible for creating this effect.

All this information is extremely relevant for visualization and how it can be used for a person to kill their body. Visualization is very similar to the placebo effect in the above example. However, visualization has the potential to produce even stronger effects. When a person is visualizing the process of themselves healing, they are sending their brain some powerful messages that instruct it to produce chemical compounds that help begin the healing process. The main roadblock here is that a person needs to be able to back up their visualization with strong self-belief that they can make this process work. That, unfortunately, is never a guarantee. However, simply focusing visualization on the person's body in a specific way helps them focus their energy, which will begin to start the healing process.

In this technique, we will be focusing on three ways that you can use visualization for the purpose of healing.

The Earth Energy Visualization

This technique requires you to close your eyes, either sitting down or standing up and allowing yourself to be grounded to the Earth. Simply visualize the energy of the earth passing through your body and healing it as it travels. You can also use this visualization by holding on to nature, like a large tree trunk, and drawing upon its earthly energy.

The Golden Ball Visualization

The second technique requires you to sit in a quiet place and begin to visualize a golden ball of light or energy that begins to surround your body. This energy starts off as a small speck within your heart—and with every inhale and exhale, it begins to grow and expand until your entire body is enveloped. You begin first to feel its healing properties as you imagine the light to work through your body and allow it to travel through your veins.

The Fireball Visualization

This last technique has the purpose of helping a person to manage their pain more effectively. In this visualization, you will sit quietly with your eyes shut and begin to focus on an area of your body where you feel pain or discomfort. Visualize that painful area as a red, big, and bright fireball. Then, with every breath you begin to take the fireball in that area begins to shrink smaller and smaller until it becomes a tiny speck on your body. As the fireball shrinks, imagine the pain that you are feeling begins melting away like snow on a warm day.

Feel free to use the techniques altogether or explore them individually. There are numerous other visualization methods that can be used for internal and external healing processes. There are numerous visualizations up there that you can try and explore until you find the one that works best for your individual self.

Chapter 8: How to Use Meditation to Achieve Your Goals

One of the most powerful and inspiring things that humans can do is being able to visualize the things that they want to manifest and then actually making it happen. The power of the human mind is extraordinary, especially when it is coupled with mindfulness practices like meditation. Using meditation, a person can increase their ability and make heaps of progress towards the life that they want to create for themselves.

Goal setting is the first action that a person needs to make in order to reach their goals. The purpose behind setting a goal is so that a person would be able to achieve their desired results. When a goal is set carefully with focus, momentum, action, and intention, setting and achieving goals is the first step that a person needs to take in order to move from where they are now to where they want to be. However, they need to know where it is that they want to be—the "where" begins with the person envisioning it.

The first step to this is to start with imagining the end in mind and work backward (this is what we discussed in the visualization chapter). Many people mistake their goal for their vision—when the goal is actually the final result. They will set a goal without thinking about what the goal will allow them to do, be, or have in the long term. For a person to make the most out of their goal-setting process, it is important to think about what quality of lifestyle they would want to achieve ultimately. For the purpose of clarity, let's talk a little bit more about the difference between a person's vision and their goal.

Your Vision vs. Your Goal

A person's vision isn't something that needs to be created from scratch; in fact, it is something that already exists inside them. They simply need to get in touch with it. A person's vision is the big picture of their desired outcomes. It represents the most important things to that person and is often compelling, inspiring, exciting, and filled with many positive emotions.

A goal, on the other hand, is different. A goal is very specifically designed that requires tasks that need to be completed in order to get to the thing that they want at the end of their journey. The downside here is that a person's goal may not initiate those positive emotions that become an inspiration. Goals act more like steppingstones on a path that will lead you to your ultimate end goal.

The most popular and effective way to build your goals is using the SMART goals format. You may have done or heard of this before at your workplace or while you were in school. SMART stands for specific, measurable, achievable, resources, and time. This helps you make sure that your goals are specific and concise, you have a way of measuring them, they are goals that are achievable, you have or have a way of getting the necessary resources, and you have a timeline in which you want your goals to be met.

By using imagery that is vivid and highly detailed, it is a very powerful way for someone to train their mind to go after the things that they want. Remember the time when we discussed how athletes often use visualization to help themselves train? For example, famous golf athlete Tiger Woods has been using visualization to help train his golfing techniques ever since he was a teenager. Even the NBA star Michael Jordan used mental imagery to help get himself into the mindset that he wants to be in order to make his famous three-point shots. If professional athletes use visualization techniques, they can enhance their ability to be the best. You can also use visualization and meditation to help you achieve your goals.

Ten Steps of Meditating to Help You Achieve Your Goals

In this ten-step guide, we will be using a mix of visualization and meditation to guide you into focusing on your goals. This is very similar to what we learned with visualization; researchers have found that by visualizing and meditating to the process of a person achieving their goals, it will help them to do it in real life. Try these following steps of guided meditation to help put your goal into the future:

1. Start by thinking of an area of your life in your mind. Choose something where you have been struggling with, or you would like to change.

2. Now, start to imagine the best possible outcome that you would like to be living in with regards to the area that you've selected. Imagine this, 6 to 12 months from now. What is the reality that you are looking to achieve? Try not to get caught up with any negativity or limitations; instead, just allow yourself to imagine and get carried away with your strongest goals.

3. Focus your mind on connecting with just one goal that you would like to achieve over the next three months. Make sure your goal is a good one and is as meaningful as possible. If you choose a goal that isn't meaningful or doesn't hold a lot of weight, the final result won't feel special for you. Make sure to choose something that is significant enough so that once you achieve this goal, you will feel a high sense of accomplishment and

motivation for your next goal. Be sure to run your goal through the SMART acronym to ensure that it is a goal that is set up for success.

4. Now that you are starting to feel connected with the goal that you've set, try to imagine what your life will be like once you achieve the goal. Visualize a picture or movie in your mind and try to view it as if you are looking at it through your own pair of eyes. Factor in all the other sensory perceptions to try to imagine the most real and positive feelings. Where are you? Who is with you? What are the things happening around you?

5. Now, begin to step out of the picture or movie that you've imagined and begin to imagine yourself floating up in the air above where you are sitting now while taking that imagery with you. Take a deep breath and as you breathe out, use your breath to give life to the image and fill it with intention and positive energy. Repeat this five times.

6. In this step, it is time to imagine yourself floating out into the future while imagining yourself dropping the imagery that you've created for your goal down into your real-life below you at the exact time and date that you've set for yourself to reach this goal.

7. Pay attention to all the things that need to happen between then and now and how it is beginning to re-evaluate itself in order to support you in achieving that goal. Visualize this process and all those events to make it feel as realistic as possible.

8. Once you feel like that step is complete, bring your awareness back to the present, and with your eyes still shut, start to think about what steps you will need to

take in the next few days that will help you move closer to achieving your goal.

9. Take a few more deep breaths in order to ground yourself to the present before opening your eyes. Now, before you forget, write down a list of steps that you need to take in order to achieve your goal or begin to write down your experience in your journal so that you don't forget.

10. In this last step, you will focus on taking action and staying focused. Make sure that you are doing something that brings you closer to achieving your goal daily.

Use this meditation and visualization technique once a week after you first complete the steps. By doing so, it helps you continue to move forward towards your end goal and help you bring your vision into real life. Seeing is believing, so through using your mind and meditation, you can create the best future that you have imagined for yourself.

Chapter 9: Self-Disciplined People Are Successful People

At this point in the book, you have learned everything—from what self-discipline is all the way to utilizing visualization at meditation to help improve it. There are many famous people who have had such strong self-discipline despite the obstacles and challenges that they encountered throughout their journey but still found their way to achieving their goals and finding success. In this chapter, we will be learning about the success stories of a few famous people who, despite all the odds that were stacked against them, found a way to achieve their goal through pure self-discipline and determination. We will be learning about the stories of Bill Gates, Steve Jobs, and Oprah Winfrey. Throughout these stories, I will try to highlight the parts and the actions where these people exercise self-discipline in order to overcome obstacles. The stories of these people are meant to help you get a real-life example of how people can exercise self-discipline to reach their goals even if their goals seem to be too big or too far-fetched.

The Story of Bill Gates

So, let's begin with the story of Bill Gates. Almost everybody on this planet knows of Bill Gates and his creation of the most popular and widely used computer platform in the world—Microsoft. For those of you who don't know him, I will give a brief introduction on who Bill Gates is. Bill Gates is an entrepreneur and businessman, and he and his partner Paul Allen founded and built Microsoft, which is the world's largest software business through good business and aggressive business strategy. Due to this, Bill Gates became one of the richest people in the world. However, in 2014, Bill Gates announced that he would be stepping down as the chairman of Microsoft in order to focus more on his passion, which is his foundation—the Bill and Melinda Gates Foundation.

Bill Gates grew up in a family where the atmosphere has always been warm. All three of the Gates children were constantly encouraged to strive for excellence and to be competitive. This environment built by his parents is one that Fosters encouragement and acknowledgment, which is required for children to grow up with the right self-esteem. This is important to know because, without self-esteem, it is easier for a person to lack self-discipline as they are unable to believe in their own worth and actions. Bill Gates showed very early signs of competitiveness when he organized family games during their summer vacations. He also loved playing board games like Risk and was extremely good at Monopoly. Bill Gates was also very close to his mother as she devoted most of her time after her teaching career to raise her children and work with numerous charities. She often would take Bill Gates along with her when she volunteered within her community and local schools.

Bill Gates was also a very intellectually curious individual. He spent many hours reading informative books like the encyclopedia. When he was around the age of 12, his parents began to have slight concerns about his behavior. He was doing extremely well in school but seemed to be withdrawn and board most of the time, and his parents worried that he might become a loner. Even though Bill Gates' parents were big fans of public education, they enrolled Bill into a private school when he turned 13 as they felt that he was not being challenged enough. He excelled in nearly all his subjects but showed a lot of interest and dedication when it came to computer classes. Bill Gates began to become very passionate about all the things a computer was capable of and spent most of his free time working on a computer.

Now, here comes one of the most well-known parts of Bill Gates's story. Bill Gates began school at Harvard University in 1973, originally with the intention that he was going to have a career in law. Much to his parents' dismay, Bill Gates ended up dropping out of Harvard in 1975 to start his own business, Microsoft. In 1975, Bill Gates and his partner Paul Allen officially formed Microsoft. At first, their business was not smooth sailing. Although the first product that they have ever created for Microsoft broke even with their company fees and they were making royalties, it wasn't exactly meeting their overhead. He later found out that only about 10% of the people that were using his software paid for it. Although Microsoft started out as a company that was very shaky, by 1979, Microsoft was bringing in gross revenue of approximately $2.5 million dollars. At the young age of 23, Bill Gates Place himself as the CEO of the company. With his strong software development skills and intelligent sense of business, he let the company and personally reviewed every line of code that the Microsoft products offered.

You can see that there are multiple instances and Bill Gates's story of creating Microsoft, where he was faced with many challenges and obstacles. There were parts of his story where Bill Gates did not have support from his family, yet his vision of his company and what he could do was strong enough to help them overcome the negative judgments and challenges that were thrown in his way. If Bill Gates had given up during the first obstacle he had encountered, Microsoft would not exist today. In addition, if Bill Gates had decided to stay at Harvard and continue pursuing his degree in law, even though that was not what he was passionate about, we would also not have Microsoft today. I hope that throughout the story, you can see the themes of self-discipline that Bill Gates exercised over his early career. He likely had a strong visualization of his successful company Microsoft and created the steps that he needed to take for himself in order to get to that goal. By doing this, Microsoft became a reality and not just a goal that he has imagined in his mind.

The Story of Steve Jobs

In our next story, we will learn about the famous Steve Jobs and how he came to build Apple. Just like Bill Gates, almost everyone on this planet knows who he is and likely owns one of his products. For those who don't, I will give a brief introduction to Steve Jobs. Steve Jobs was an entrepreneur and an American inventor and designer. He was the co-founder, chief executive, and chairman of Apple computer. Apple is a cutting-edge technology company that has invented some of the most revolutionary products today that include the iPod, iPhone, and iPad.

Steve Jobs was born in 1955, and his biological parents were to graduate students of the University of Wisconsin who gave him up for adoption. Steve was adopted by Clara and Paul Jobs when he was an infant. His mother worked as an accountant, and his father was a machinist and a coast guard veteran. Steve lived with his adoptive family in Mountain View, California, which would later become the famous Silicon Valley. In Steve Jobs' childhood, he and his father would work with many electronics in their family garage. His father showed him how to take apart and rebuild Electronics, which was a hobby that helped build tenacity and confidence in the young Steve Jobs. Just like Bill Gates, Steve Jobs also had a childhood where his parents were encouraging and instilled confidence in him. This led to him having healthy self-esteem later in adulthood, which is an important prerequisite for having strong self-discipline.

While Steve Jobs was always a very innovative thinker and intelligent boy, his youth was full of frustrations when it came to formal schooling. Steve Jobs was a big prankster during his time in elementary school due to his boredom. His teacher in fourth grade often had to bribe him to get him to study. However, Steve Jobs tested so well that the school administrators wanted him to skip grades and go straight to high school. This was a proposal that his parents had declined. After Steve Jobs graduated high school, he enrolled at Reed College in Portland, Oregon. However, Steve Jobs still lacked a lot of direction, and he ended up dropping out of college after the first six months and spent the next year-and-a-half dropping in on creative classes that were offered at the school. In 1974, Steve Jobs took a job as a video game designer with Atari. However, several months later, he quit his job in order to search for spiritual enlightenment in India, where he traveled for many months and experimented with psychedelic drugs.

In 1976, when Steve Jobs was only 21 years old, he and his partner Steve Wozniak started the company Apple Computer in Steve Jobs' family garage. They funded the jumpstart of their company through jobs selling his Volkswagen bus and Wozniak selling his scientific calculator. Steve Jobs and Steve Wozniak built Apple computers with the goal of wanting to democratize technology and make computers smaller, more intuitive, cheaper, and more accessible to everyday consumers.

Steve Jobs and Steve Wozniak created a series of personal computers that were user-friendly and initially marketed the computers for around $600 each. The first generation of Apple computers made the company around $800,000.

Three years later, when they release the second model of the Apple computer, their company's sales increased to 139 million dollars, which is about a 700% increase. In 1980, Apple Computer became a public traded company with a value of 1.2 billion dollars by its first day of trading. However, the next several products that Apple release had many design flaws, which resulted in numerous recalls and a lot of consumer disappointment. IBM began to surpass Apple and sales, and now, Apple had to compete in a business world that is dominated by PC and IBM.

In 1984, Apple released the first Macintosh, which was marketed as a computer that has the lifestyle of romance, youth, and creativity. Despite the increased and positive sales and a performance that is much superior to IBM's computers, the Macintosh was still not compatible with IBM. Steve Jobs' CEO believed that he was hurting Apple, and the executives started to drive him out of business. Since Steve Jobs did not actually have an official title within the company that he had founded, Steve was pushed into a marginalized position and then left Apple in 1985.

However, in 1997, Steve Jobs returned to Apple as the CEO. He began to redo a lot of things within his company, and he is famously credited with rebuilding the company in the 1990s. Steve Jobs built a new management team and altered its stock options and was able to put Apple back on track. His famous invention of products like the iMac accomplished with strong branding campaigns and stylish designs began to become popular within the consumer base once again. Over the next few years, Apple created revolutionary products like the iPod, iPhone, and MacBook Air, which their competitors immediately scrambled whenever Apple released a new product in order to create technologies that were comparable.

By 2007, the stocks at Apple were worth almost $200 a share, and the company brought in a huge $1.58-billion-dollar profit.

Throughout the story of Steve Jobs, you can see multiple instances where he faced difficult obstacles and hardships like when he was phased out of his own company back in 1984. However, despite the time that Steve Jobs took away from Apple, he never gave up on the company that he has envisioned for so long and got himself back on track to create one of the most successful companies in the world today. This is just what self-discipline is. The journey to success in achieving the goals that are most important to you will never be a straight line. There will be many obstacles along the way, some of which may take many years to overcome, but the important theme in this is that you should never give up on the goal that you've envisioned for yourself. If Steve Jobs gave up on his goal after he was phased out from his own company, we would not have the revolutionary Apple products that we have today.

The Story of Oprah Winfrey

Oprah Winfrey is a globally famous talk show host, actress, media executive, and billionaire. Just like Bill Gates and Steve Jobs, almost everyone on the planet knows of Oprah Winfrey. For those who don't know who she is, I will give a brief introduction. Oprah Winfrey is the most famous for being the host of her incredibly popular show—The Oprah Winfrey Show.

Oprah was born in a small town in Mississippi in 1954. Unlike Steve Jobs and Bill Gates, she had a very troubled adolescence, where she was sexually abused by numerous friends of her mother and several her male relatives. After that, Oprah moved to Nashville to live with her father, who was a businessman and a barber. Oprah was enrolled at

Tennessee State University in 1971 and began working in radio and television Broadcasting. After her schooling, in 1976, Oprah moved to Baltimore, Maryland, where she began hosting a TV show called people are talking. The show quickly became a hit, and Oprah stayed as a host for eight years until she was recruited by the Chicago TV station to host A.M. Chicago, which was her own morning show. Her biggest competitor at the time was Phil Donahue. However, within several months of her own show, Oprah's warm-hearted personal style and openness had gained her 100000 more viewers than Phil Donahue, which took her Show from the last place to first place in the ratings.

In 1986, Oprah Winfrey launched her own show, the Oprah Winfrey show. It was aired on 120 channels and an audience of over 10 million people. By the end of its first year, the show grossed 125 million dollars. She also then gained ownership of the program from ABC and gave it to her own production company, Harpo Productions. She began to make more and more money due to this business decision.

Oprah Winfrey has struggled with her weight publicly and has many well-documented Weight Loss efforts. Between the late 80s and the late 90s, her weight fluctuated based on whatever diet and exercise she was doing. After numerous attempts, she was able to reach a weight that she was happy with, and she even bought a 10% stake in the company Weight Watchers. She became an advisor for the company and appeared on TV as she acted as the spokesperson as well. Although Weight Watchers had been in a big funk for a while, Oprah's help revived the company, and it saw an increase in stock prices and membership.

Throughout the life story of Oprah Winfrey, you can see that she had a very troubled childhood but still had enough self-discipline to get herself back on her feet to pursue a career that would soon make her billions of dollars. Until this day, she is still one of the most famous and successful African American women. If she had given up at the first few obstacles that life had thrown in her way, she would not be where she is today. Since her success, she has millions of dollars to various charities and causes.

Conclusion

At this point, you have gotten to the end of the book. Congratulations on having the self-discipline to finish an entire book teaching you about self-discipline. Let's do a quick recap of everything we've learned far. We started off with the basic but important topics of what self-discipline is, why it's important, and what a person can achieve through self-discipline. We then drove a little deeper into self-discipline and learned about the psychology behind it. We spoke a lot about willpower and discussed whether it is a limited or unlimited resource or not. We learned that willpower is something that strongly drives self-discipline and that a person with more willpower is likely to be able to withstand temptation, while someone with low willpower might not be strong enough to resist when temptation comes their way.

We also dove into the details of the benefits and drawbacks that come with strengthening self-discipline. We learned that self-discipline could bring benefits that improve a person's inner strength and character, allow them to withstand temptation, heighten their chances of success, help them build better relationships, and help them feel less offended. After that, you learned the different causes of low self-discipline, as well as a couple of tips on what you can do to mitigate that. We then moved on to the more instruction-based portion of this book, where we focused on why self-discipline is the key to success and the 10 steps that a person can take to achieve self-discipline. Within those 10 steps, you learned that you must understand your weaknesses and then remove temptation based on what your weaknesses are. We discussed how setting clear goals and having a plan is crucial to building self-discipline. More physical things like eating healthily and eating often and rewarding yourself are important in the process of using self-discipline. Since it has been proven that a person's brain is energized through glucose consumption if a person is hungry or is having low blood sugar, it makes it very hard for them to resist temptation or even stay focused, in general.

You were then provided with a few tips and habits that a person can use in order to build their self-discipline. You learned that building gratitude, forgiveness, meditation, active goal setting, sleep, exercise, organization, time management, and persistence played a huge role in self-discipline. In the chapter after that, you learned about some of the challenges of self-discipline so that you can start preparing to overcome these obstacles as you face them. We then moved on to learning two methods that can help a person increase their self-discipline. We learned how to use visualization and meditation to achieve our goals. We learned that visualization had been proven to be almost or just as effective as practicing the action of something itself. We then ended off the book by learning some stories of famous people that have exercised self-discipline in order to achieve their goals. We learned the stories of Bill Gates, Steve Jobs, and Oprah Winfrey. One common theme throughout all three of their life stories is that no matter how many and how big the obstacles that they faced; their self-discipline pushes them through to success.

Hence, with all this new information that you just learned, what's next for you? Keep in mind that self-discipline is all about setting goals, breaking them down into smaller ones, and disciplining yourself so that those smaller and daily goals become a part of your everyday routine. When you complete the tasks related to achieving your goal becomes a habit that is a part of your life, *that* is when you no longer need to draw into your willpower resources to exercise that action. By doing this, it will leave you more energy to start incorporating other actions of other goals that you would like to achieve. Like I mentioned throughout this book, think of an important goal that you have in mind and work backward and break it down into smaller ones. Start small, and don't give up no matter the obstacles that come your way. I hope that one of the takeaways that you got from this book is that there will always be numerous challenges and obstacles in life. Just like Bill Gates, Steve Jobs, and Oprah Winfrey, they overcame large challenges no matter how much time it took them to be able to move past them. At the end of it all, they all achieved the greatest reward of all, which is accomplishing their life goals.

Consistency really is the key when it comes to self-discipline. Always remember that bad habits take years to build, which means that it will also take years to break them down. Rebuilding good habits takes just as long. If you find yourself falling into temptation or find that it's getting harder and harder to draw from your willpower resources to continue to do the actions that you promised yourself that you would do, try to think about the purpose behind your goal. If you've learned something from this book, one of the things may probably be that a meaningful goal creates more motivation than a goal without substance. Whenever you feel yourself losing motivation or feeling like you're unable to resist temptation, think about what motivates you in the first place to go after that goal. Lastly, I wish you the best in your journey of self-discipline! Remember to forgive yourself if you have any lapses on your journey, and always keep moving forward.

Improve Your Social Skills

The ultimate training guide for enhancing your social skills and self-esteem and for living a successful life becoming the best version of yourself.

Jack Gilman

Introduction

Congratulations on purchasing *Improve Your Social Skills.* Being able to socialize through effective communication skills is an important life skill. It gives us the opportunity to pass information to the people we are connecting with and understand what is said to us. Building sustainable relationships can help us interact with people as well as reduce anxiety and stress in our lives. In fact, social skills are linked to improved mental health since having great friends, and close relations can "buffer" us from feeling moody and anxious. Thus, we rely on social skills to have functional personal and professional life through effective socialization.

In this book, you will have an overview of the key social skills that are crucial for every interaction. You will learn about key social skills, including listening, which is a fundamental skill for conversation, empathy, verbal and nonverbal communication, cooperation, and making eye contact. You will also get to learn the science of holding conversation, including how to start and end a conversation successfully and keep going with the story. You will also learn about the types of social skills deficits and their effects on an individual. Further, you understand what it means to lack social skills, and how this can affect your relationship with other people. Improve Your Social Skills also covers the strategies to react to different body languages and what different gestures mean in a conversation.

While there are plenty of books highlighting the significance of social skills in communication, you've decided to choose this specific one and we thank you for that! Enjoy your read!

Chapter 1: Introduction to Social Skills

An important part of growing up is to learn how to communicate, behave around, and understand other people. Having knowledge of such skills is necessary in order to have a better relationship with others and cope in society. We must know how to start conversations, learn conventions and gestures, what is to be said in a particular context, what not to be said, how to greet others, and how best to interact with fellow human beings. Thus, most part of growing up involves acquiring social skills that can enhance our connection with other people.

What Are Social Skills

There are several definitions of social skills. In general, it refers to any skill that facilitates communication and interaction with others. This includes establishing an appropriate eye contact, careful listening, appropriately beginning an interaction, turn-taking, being aware of other people's feelings, interpreting and using non-verbal communication, and knowing how to close conversation.

The concept has also been defined by different theorists in terms of the behavior of individuals. As such, it means "the type of behaviors that are basic to a successful face-to-face communication among individuals." Some scientists have also extended the definition to include the goals of individuals, claiming that it refers to "social behaviors, which are effective in achieving the goals of the people who interact."

Considering the above definition, social skills:

- Are acquire through learning;

- Entails discrete, specific verbal and non-verbal

behaviors;

- Comprises of effective initiations and responses;

- Maximize social reinforcement from those people one interacts with;

- Need appropriate timing, and are interactive in nature;

- Are influenced by different factors, including sex, age, and a person's status

Social skills should be appropriate in every situation. An individual who has social skills would adapt his behaviors in order to meet the needs of individuals that he/she shares a particular social context. This means that skilled communication depends on the use of behaviorally facilitative and textually appropriate means of efficiently relating to others.

Characteristics of Social Skills

The key characteristics of social skills include:

- Social skills are goal-oriented

- Socially skilled behaviors are interrelated in that an individual may adopt more than one behavior in a particular time to achieve a goal

- Social skills are expected to be appropriate for every communication context. This means that different social skills are used for different personal and professional communication contexts

- Socially skilled behaviors involve one being judged on how socially skilled they are

- Social skills can be learned, practiced, and taught

- Social skills are cognitively controlled by an individual

Benefits of Social Skills

There are distinct benefits of having well-developed social skills, including:

More Relationships

When you identify yourself with people, you may find yourself having more friendships and even relationships. By developing social skills, you will be able to possess charisma, which is a desirable trait. People like to relate with charismatic people because they are more interesting.

Many people are unable to advance in life because they lack interpersonal relationships. By focusing on relationships, you may be able to get a job and make more friends. Effective social skills help increase happiness and satisfaction and can provide a better life outlook.

Relationships also reduce the potential negative effects of stress while also boosting self-esteem.

Enhances Communication

As you relate with other people, you automatically develop communication skills. After all, no one can have great social skills if they do not have better communication skills. Also being able to convey your ideas and thoughts may be an important skill you can develop in life.

Greater Efficiency

If you relate well with people, you will easily avoid being with those whom you don't like. Some people avoid interacting because they do not wish to spend time with those who have different interests or viewpoints from theirs. It is very easy to attend a work meeting or party if you are aware that there are at least some people who you know will be there.

If you are not interacting with particular people because they don't have common viewpoints with you, you are able to use your set of social skills to convey politely that you prefer spending time with other people.

Social Skills Enable One to Advance Career Prospects

Most professions have a "people component" and most prominent positions involve spending time interacting with colleagues, employees, and the media. It is very rare to find that a person remains isolated in the office and excel in their job positions. Many organizations prefer looking for individuals who have a particular skillset and have the ability to work well with a team and motivate others.

Increased Overall Happiness

Getting along with other people and understanding others can open several career and person-related doors. If you are able to confidently begin a conversation at a work conference, you may land a new job opportunity with higher pay. A "hello" or a simple smile in a social gathering can lead you to form a new friendship.

Process of Learning Social Skills

There are three processes that people use to navigate the social world. These include seeing, thinking, and doing.

Seeing

Seeing involves picking up particular social cues. It refers to the process of noticing a context. You may ask yourself the following questions: Is this setting formal or casual? Are those people acquaintances or close friends? Different situations require different types of behavior. Seeing in a social situation also means noticing the behavior of other people. If you feel lost about how to act is a particular place, then you should ask yourself, "what is everyone else doing?" in order to get a hint of how to react.

Monitoring other people might also help you to change the course of things. For example, noticing that someone is bored with a story may prompt you to suggest a new topic or ask the other person what he or she would like to talk about.

Having trouble with social seeing always makes other people uncomfortable. You may do things that are not appropriate for a particular social context, like playing around when everyone is serious. Worse, you may find yourself insisting to engage in annoying or upsetting behaviors because you tend to overlook the feelings of others.

Thinking

In a social setting, thinking involves the interpretation of other people's behaviors to understand why they are engaging in such acts. Are they polite or aggressive? Are their behaviors accidental or deliberate? It also means being able to predict the likely response of other people and come up with strategies for influencing them.

Social cognition research shows that people who struggle socially always misinterpret the intentions of others. For example, people who are aggressive are more likely to view that the behavior of others stems from deliberate meanness. They are also less likely to come up with constructive strategies to address social conflicts.

Doing

In a social context, doing involves interacting with others in a positive way. Some people know what they ought to do, but they have trouble actually performing those acts. For instance, one may join a conversation, but he or she may feel anxious and end up saying nothing. Others tend to act impulsively, making inappropriate comments.

Chapter 2: Important Social Skills You Should Possess

Some essential social skills significantly contribute to your success in life. Such social skills are not only crucial in improving your skills but could also contribute to other areas of your life, such as your health, education, spirituality, and profession.

The good news is, you can learn such social skills through training and constant practice. The following is a guide that can help you develop the social skills needed to live a very successful and contented life:

Optimism

Being optimistic in life is one of the vital social skills that can help you climb the ladder of success. Optimism works best for your personal, social, and career, and every other aspect of your life. When you stay positive, you tend to attract the attention of others, just like the way magnet works on metal. People are naturally drawn towards positive people with great optimism because the attitude makes them feel good about themselves and life in general. On the other hand, negative energy tends to draw people far away from you.

You, therefore, need to go about your daily activities with an upbeat and energetic way while wearing that big smile that tells others you are the most optimistic person around them. If you go about your work while complaining and nagging about how unfair life is or how your bosses are so insensitive to your needs, the consequence is that people will tend to snap at you for always being in a terrible mood.

You need to foster your optimism by paying close attention to your thoughts. Monitor your thoughts and remove the negative while you strive to nurture the positive thoughts. Thoughts eventually become feelings which, in turn, will give birth to actions or behaviors. You, therefore, need to remove the root of your negativity by completely blocking any negative thought from entering your mind. Strive to replace any negative thoughts with positive ones instead.

Alternatively, you can nourish your positivity by staying around people who have a positive attitude toward life. Such people are upbeat about what life has to offer, whether it is negative or not.

Compassion

Compassion means being deeply aware of the suffering of others with a sincere hope that they will get appropriate relief soon. The skill of being compassionate allows you to identify and feel other people's pain naturally. It also brings a desire for you to help them out of their misery.

If you wish to be compassionate, then you must be willing to learn how to be an attentive listener. Listen carefully as others are narrating their problems to you. You should also try to relate their problems by describing any similar situation which you faced in the past. You can then try to help them by sharing how you solved the past problem which you faced. You can also assist them by coming up with new solutions to the issues they are facing.

You can also get involved with the sufferer through charity work such as the red cross or by volunteering your services to help them. For example, if you are a doctor, you can volunteer your services by helping victims of accidents or any other natural calamity.

Politeness

Your parents or guardians must have insisted on being polite as part of good manners from the time you were a young child. This skill is crucial from then up to date. Being polite could be the difference between being a successful person in life or a sour looser. Nobody wants to associate with an arrogant person who is seeking for their self-inflated ego to be massaged. This is why no matter your standing in society, you should always line when someone is in front of you.

The social skill of politeness can be learned and fostered over time. You should make conscious efforts to watch what you say to others whenever you are conversing. Choose the words you use in conversation carefully and always think twice before you say them to avoid negative words or emotions from leaving your lips.

Always use polite words like "thank you, I am sorry, excuse me, or please" whenever you are addressing other people. It will not only tell them that you are polite but will also enable them to develop a definite liking for you.

Ensure you get into the habit of being polite always to be socially accepted by others.

Emotional Intelligence

When you are emotionally intelligent, then you know how to act, what to say, or how to react as every situation demands. Emotionally intelligent people are also sensitive to the emotions of others. For example, the choice of words you use in a party is quite different from the ones you use at a funeral.

Emotional intelligence is also about how you manage your own emotions and how you react to the feelings of others. If you possess this critical social skill, then you are ahead in the skills necessary to manage conflicts. You are also at an advantage in how well you respond to the needs of others. Emotional intelligence also empowers you to control your own emotions so as not to let them overflow and disrupt your life.

You can nurture this skill by being aware of your feelings at all times. Self-awareness means having an accurate assessment of what exactly you are capable of when subjected to a demanding situation. You should also be mindful of when you need help from others and what usually triggers off your emotions.

Discipline

Being disciplined means you behave in a manner acceptable to society. It means your behavior must be per the societal rules, customs, laws, policies, or any other guideline. When you are disciplined, then you willingly comply with the systematic method of a given environment. You exercise self-control that makes you an acceptable person in society.

You can nurture self-discipline by treating yourself with appropriate rewards every time you succeed in doing something right. You should not wait for the prompting of others to be disciplined, be self-driven in going for your dreams and desires. You should also make the necessary changes to your routine, get rid of undesirable behaviors, and strive to push yourself harder towards your goals. You also need to get out of your comfort zone and go for new targets.

Diligence

The famous saying is that diligence is the mother of all good luck. And this is actually true. If you want to achieve credibility in whatever you are doing, then you should always give your work due diligence. Diligence enables people to appreciate their hard work. It is a virtue that wins the hearts and praise of others.

You can foster this critical skill by avoiding any short cuts in whatever you are engaged in. Acknowledge the fact that life has no shortcuts, and nothing comes easy, and therefore, you need to roll up your sleeves and get dirty to achieve your dreams. You can choose to track your diligence by keeping a journal in which you record the daily tasks which you have accomplished and which will contribute to your long-term goals. You should aim at achieving at least two tasks each day.

Patience

Patience is another fundamental social skill you should possess. Being patient with yourself and, most importantly, with others is the key to having a fruitful life. Most of the nuisances you face in your daily life come from other people. For example, if you find yourself stuck on traffic, it could be because someone failed to observe the traffic rules, causing inconveniences to every other road user. If you are late at the meeting a deadline, it could be because a team member has been overly slow at getting their part of the work done on time. Human error and mistakes are entirely natural, so you should avoid blaming others unnecessarily whenever an issue occurs.

You can foster this critical social skill by practicing meditative techniques. For example, before you get angry at everyone, and start blaming them for your mistakes, take a moment to reflect on what is making you so mad. Once you have identified what is triggering your anger, close your eyes, and take three deep breathes. You should count from1 up to 10 as you do this. If you learn this skill well, then you will react most sensibly and constructively the next time you are faced with a similar situation.

Affability

Another important social skill to possess is practicing the quality of being affable. An affable person is one who is friendly, amiable, or pleasant. If you are an affable person, then others find it easy to approach and talk to you because they find you quite welcoming and friendly.

You need to learn how to get well with everyone, no matter their standing in life, their status, or their opinions. You should be friendly enough to mingle and interact with others freely as you laugh and share anything concerning life.

As a social person, you must have cultivated strong friendships with others in the course of your interaction. These are real friends who won't think twice at lending their helping hand whenever you are faced with a challenge. You should, therefore, learn to value and treat everyone well, even the random stranger you share a train ride with as you go to work. You never know when such persons come in handy later on in your life.

You can foster this skill by interacting with people wherever and whenever possible. Be the first to break the ice the next time you are sitting next to that stranger in public. Learn to engage the people around you in lively conversations; be it when you meet them at the church, restaurant, bus station, or train. You can do this by complimenting them or asking relevant questions, for example, asking about time. Once they respond, you should listen attentively with a lot of interest.

Be a Good Listener

They say successful people listen more and talk less, and how true this is. You should learn to pay attention to what others are saying. Show your interest in what the other person is telling you. Listening carefully to what others are saying without interrupting them unnecessarily. If you must interrupt them, then do so at an appropriate time, not when they are in the middle of a sentence. Listening skills also mean you learn the practice of good turn-taking. You should know when to speak and when to let the other person talk. Failure to listen carefully means you won't be able to learn or exchange information with others.

You can foster this vital skill by consistently practicing turn-taking habits. For example, avoid dominating a discussion as you interact with others. Allow others to contribute to the conversation. Be sensitive to the amount of input you are giving to a conversation as compared to theirs.

If you notice your input to a conversation is above 80 %, then you need to keep quiet and allow others to give their information too.

Forgiveness

Practicing forgiveness whenever others wrong you, is crucial to your happiness and overall wellbeing. Forgiving others means you completely erase the pain and bitterness you feel towards them for the wrongs they did to you willingly or unwillingly. A forgiving heart is a healthy, happy, and thriving heart. You stand to gain nothing by holding on to grudges, pain, and bitterness towards your tormentors. Bearing grudges and bitterness increases stress, which will eventually harm your health. It will also reduce any possibility of making any gains through your relationship.

You need to foster forgiveness by objectively reviewing how you perceive the wrongs others did to you. Find out why they did it, was it pre-arranged or they were just carried away by the pressure of the moment. You should also determine whether you are fair in your accusations. Ask yourself whether you are unreasonable and unjust to someone who wronged you. Then put yourself in their situation. How will it feel like to hurt someone and have them forgive you of all your wrongs and vice versa?

Forgiveness doesn't make you weak in the eyes of your adversary, it actually makes you strong, so you should learn to forgive others whenever they wrong you.

Resilience

Resilience is your ability to bounce back quickly whenever a setback or a challenge hit you. If you allow yourself to be knocked down by life and you can rise again speedily and strongly, then you are a resilient person. A resilient person can adapt well in the face of a tragedy and bounce back to resume their life as if nothing terrible had happened. You should possess the power to thrive and survive, even in the most challenging environments. Whenever you fail in your endeavors, you should take it as an opportunity to start anew. Pick valuable lessons from your failure and incorporate them into your next moves.

You can learn resilience by cultivating a strong relationship with others. Always build a strong support network comprising of close friends and family who will help you overcome your challenges whenever you are faced with one.

Responsibility

Successful people are responsible for their everyday decisions and actions. They admit responsibility whenever a mistake is made. You should learn to own your problems and mistakes by taking responsibility for them. Avoid blaming your mistakes on others, especially the gullible junior workers below you. This applies even when you are not directly involved in their errors, the liability will always rest on you.

You can foster this skill by acknowledging and accepting all your responsibilities. Get to know what your responsibilities are in your place of work, at home, or even in your community. Once you have accepted your responsibilities, admit your mistakes whenever a fault is done, and take quick measures to correct it.

Leadership

They say good leaders are born, but well, they can also be made. You are probably a leader in every setting you find yourself in. It could be in a classroom setting, at the family level, or at an organizational level. To be a good leader, you need to discover your unique skills then harness your leadership skills, interests, and passion. You must also strive to lead by example by being a role model to the people you are leading. You cannot preach water and drink wine if you want to be an influential and effective leader.

Always Seek Help Whenever Necessary

Another good social skill you must develop is asking for help from others whenever you are faced with a challenge. Next time you are stuck in an unfamiliar place, don't be afraid to ask for direction from those who know the neighborhood well. This applies to classroom learning. If you don't understand a concept, reach out to others for help. You will be taken back with how people are eager to help you out of your problems.

This social skill will help improve your relationship with others because you endear yourself to the. It also tells them you are approachable and humble. Besides, even you seek help from others, and it opens many opportunities for your success.

Honesty

You should avoid giving out false, incomplete, and misleading information for self-gain. Always stick to the truth, no matter how painful it is. If you are an honest person, people will find it easy to trust you. It will also help you foster good relationships with others because, well, no one wants to hang out with a dishonest lying person.

Chapter 3: Social Skills Deficit

Social skills enable us to know how to conduct ourselves in public. However, an individual may have a social skills deficit for many reasons. It could be a lack of knowledge, or a competency issue, or an inability to acquire new skills. Sometimes it may be because of a lack of practice in the newly acquired skill or inadequate feedback. Other times, even when the skills have been taught and practiced, some internal, external factors such as anxiety, hyperactivity, or an uncomfortable environment may cause social dysfunctions in the individual. Some people generally lack social interest; therefore, their social skills remain undeveloped.

A person may not know how to behave in a particular situation, or if they possess the knowledge, they may apply it indiscriminately. For example, a person may grab a piece of cake from your hand because they may not know how to ask for it appropriately. Lack of sufficient feedback may also cause a social skills deficit, for example, a person may know specific words are profane but may not know how they affect a social situation and may, therefore, blurt them out in a gathering. To interact effectively with others, an individual must be attentive, control their impulses, and respond appropriately.

Moreover, numerous guardians hyper-plan their kids, filling their days with an excessive number of exercises- chess, football, tennis, piano, dance, school prep courses, business training, and the sky is the limit from there. We do not let youngsters set aside some effort to sit with themselves and figure out how to be social. Social aptitudes are likely the most significant things we ought to learn, and it is what we do not educate.

The initial phase in any social aptitudes preparing project ought to be to lead an exhaustive assessment of the person's present degree of social working. The evaluation should detail both the qualities and shortcomings of the individual identified with social ability. Recognition is the initial phase of taking care of social and conduct deficiencies. It is essential for you, a guardian, or instructor to work together to survey the present degree of social functioning and decide on regions that could utilize some additional assistance. Respect in all aspects of communication should be upheld as social etiquette. It means using and not abusing your communication power. The following are primary social skills deficits:

Basic Communication Skills

There are four areas that you need to excel in to be fluent in communication. These areas involve reading, writing, listening, and understanding and speaking. A proper assessment of these four areas will help you recognize your strengths and weaknesses. A basic understanding of where you are most developed and the areas you may need to put in more work.

Reading

It is not about following a string of words in a piece of writing but also the ability to comprehend the literary work to the degree intentioned by the author. It may also include graphics such as charts.

Writing

This is the ability to put down a thought in a comprehensive way for other people to read and understand. This includes poems, stories, books, and other graphic works such as drawings, pictures, icons, graphs, etc.

Listening

Listening is the ability to understand the words and non-verbal cues of the speaker. It involves reading the speaker's body language and gestures and understanding how they tie in with what they are saying. This skill of listening and understanding should be emphasized more during communication skills lessons. It forms the more substantial part of a conversation. Good listening skills are often expressed through nodding, smiling, mirroring body language, and offering feedback.

Speaking

Often, speaking is emphasized more in a communications skills class than any other skill. Speaking involves expressing yourself orally or using your body language. For example, dance is a form of "spoken" language, and it pairs well with the music. Not merely is speaking distressing, however simply, its idea is enough to deliver stomach-biting butterflies.

Speaking ranges from having an expansive diction to the ability to control your tone while using your words or gestures to enhance your communication.

Interpersonal Skills

These skills involve harmonious interactions with other people. People who do not have interpersonal skills may struggle in social contexts and may not know the appropriate responses or questions to ask to propel conversation. Some individuals may ask closed questions to control reactions and keep short discussions. Examples of interpersonal skills include active listening, dependability, responsibility, patience, motivation, leadership, etc., Interpersonal skills are most important in a workplace setting because of the interaction between colleagues. It shows you can join in an activity, wait your turn, share, and ask for permission, for example, when someone is talking.

Eye Contact

The meeting of the eyes between two people has a significant influence on social behavior. It may indicate a social and emotional exchange of information. Eye contact meaning varies widely between cultures and social circles. For example, in Japanese culture, they are taught to lower their gaze when addressing a dominant figure as a sign of respect.

Eye movement, when having a verbal or non-verbal conversation with someone, may add extra pieces of information to the subject of the matter. It is considered polite not to stare at someone that is looking at them without blinking or paying attention to anything else. It is also rude- in the Western culture- not to look someone in the eye when you are talking to them, or them you. Eye contact is an incredibly expressional form of social interaction.

Empathy

The ability to share the feelings of others is a useful social skill. Understanding these feelings and creating a harmonious relationship with other people builds a rapport. These skills, however, may be impeded by the lack of particular cognitive and behavioral abilities such as anxiety and autism. People who suffer from autistic strains also suffer from social impairment.

These people tend to focus either more on themselves and their inadequacies and are unable to give other people the attention they require for a conversation to take place. Or, they may focus on other people and please them to avoid confrontations. Others shut down in social environments. You can ask yourself the following questions, among others, to find out if you are good at showing empathy and building rapport:

- Do I care about what the other person has to say?

- Do I put myself in their shoes when I listen to what they are saying?

- I like to tell people that I know exactly what they feel- but do I? Is it appropriate to tell them this?

- Do I compete with other people's stories by telling them about my experiences?

Cultivation of emotional intelligence helps you with emotional fluency and rapport.

Problem-Solving

This skill involves critical thinking, decision-making, seeking help, and thanking others for their support, as well as apologizing when you are wrong. Critical thinking is the way of seeing what is happening in your environment; distinguishing things that could be changed or improved; diagnosing why the present state is how it is, and the variables and powers that impact it; creating methodologies and choices to influence change; settling on choices about which decision to make; making a move to execute the changes; and watching the effect of those activities in nature.

Problem-solving ties in with other communication skills such as listening and interpersonal skills. A person may struggle with confrontation and therefore choose to avoid it as opposed to confronting the problem and seeking to solve it, bringing about poor conflict resolution.

While some people may grapple with being sore losers, others have trouble with understanding the root of a problem, therefore, may lack the know-how to solve it. Solving problems is the entire foundation of the evolution theory. Critical thinking is significant both to people and organizations since it empowers us to apply authority over our environment.

Cooperation

This is the ability to work together. It fosters a stable corporate relationship and personal relationships. When the parties have common interests that overlap, a need to work together to accomplish these desires is born. Cooperation should never be coerced or unintentional; it should always be voluntary. Communication helps people band together and cooperate.

Competition

People sometimes interact in a competition for control of resources. Competition is the inverse of cooperation because if the underlying interests do not agree, then strive for power is the next solution. Charles Darwin put it so eloquently when he said, "the species that survives is not always the strongest, but the most adaptable to change." Competition is an innate characteristic in all living organisms. Competition drove us to not only biological evolution but also economic development.

However, competition can also be used as a pastime; for example, in sports, that is why it is necessary to refine your social skills during such interactions.

Personal Space

Many people respect the psychological ownership of the area in their immediate surroundings. However, some people violate personal space by coming too close to other people "getting in their space." In some primitive cultures and environments such as the wilderness, invasion of personal space is seen as an act of aggression and an invitation to fight.

With permission, however, encroaching on personal space shows how you relate to the other person. The sense of personal space is closely tied to the relationship between individuals. Therefore, if you do not know someone very well, it may be safer for both of you to maintain a respectable distance between yourselves for the sake of healthy interaction.

Accountability

Accountability is being mature enough to accept responsibility or answerability for your actions. For example, if you accidentally poison your friend's dog with a small piece of chocolate, it is the responsible thing to do to come forward and accept blame for the dog's illness.

Effective practice and training programs are needed to develop the social skills to a fluent level. We begin to develop these skills at infancy as we interact with our parents, other children at daycares, and even at the playgrounds. The different developmental milestones shape our long-term social-behavioral skills.

Body Language and Non-Verbal Cues

Weak body expressions lead to poor communication. Most of the communication happens non-verbally; researchers say between 60-70 percent of all communication. What's more, we converse with our bodies without even realizing it. For example, when you are in a public area, and you cross your arms, that gesture shows apprehensiveness or guarding yourself and hunched over shoulders show an inferiority complex.

Another commonly notable expression of body language is flirting. Although most people are not able to "read" flirtatious body language, they can express themselves in this way-willingly or unwillingly. For example, leaning into the conversation, open body stance, brief light contact, smiling and nodding, playfulness with your hands and mouth, etc.

Clothing is another non-verbal cue that is quite vivid, although often overlooked. That is why there is an appropriate dress code for specific functions. For example, a tux is suitable for men's wear for a wedding and formal feast, while bathing suits are appropriate for the beach. When you wear a sweater to the beach, you may be ill or sending the wrong message to everyone else on that beach. Consider how emos or hipsters dress because they are sending a message on how they want the world to view them.

Stereotypes

When most people fall into stereotypical groups, some do not. The social skill deficit here applies when you have a preconceived notion about everyone who seems to belong to a particular group. But because we are social beings, the amount of information our brains receive from our environments may be too much to be finely processed; however, our brain compartmentalizes information for faster processing.

With the grouping of information to form stereotypes, prejudice is likely to occur. For example, African American males are considered a danger to society because recent history suggests that a few bad apples have been a menace to society. Prejudice may lead to wrong conclusions and creates an "us" versus "them" mentality.

This way of thinking creates cognitive opposition between two distinct social groups of people, the in-groups, and the outcasts- the rest. This opposition may lead to mistreatment of the outgroup. For example, the holocaust is an outstanding demonstration of stereotyping gone colossally wrong.

Poor Social Skills and How They Affect an Individual

Struggling with social situations may pose a mental and physical hazard to an individual. This is because when you are unsure of how to interact with other people, you feel lonelier and more removed from society, which may cause stress or anxiety. It is common knowledge that cognitive and psychological challenges may create a social skills deficit, but we only recently correlated poor social skills to affect the quality of life.

Deficiency in social skills does not affect only the individuals with it, but also their partners at work, or in personal and family lives. However, most people who lack social skills are usually unaware of their problem, let alone how to solve it. The frantic search for meaningful relationships goes on forever, increasing mental anguish. Society continues to disregard the distress in these people mainly because it cannot be explicitly identified or addressed.

Technology, while it may have its advantages, also poses a threat to the development of social skills in heavy users. Especially children exposed to technology and the influences of social media at a tender age, they may experience some delayed social developmental issues.

Sensory Processing

The brain may have trouble processing all the stimulus it is receiving from a social environment; therefore, the individual suffering from social skills deficiency may not understand their environment or what is required of them in certain situations.

Reasoning

The ability to reason makes you able to solve problems. Therefore, when your brain fails to organize the sensory information it is receiving, it fails you when you need to understand and sort out a situation. Reasoning is an invaluable ability that every human being needs to develop.

Behavior

When someone has a social skills deficit, they may also experience difficulties in response. They may not know how to conduct themselves in a stimulating environment or how their behavior may affect other people.

Performance

When someone is intellectually gifted but is challenged in basic communication skills, they may not be able to express themselves adequately. This inability may cause a decline in performance. They may misinterpret literary works, or spoken language, or not be able to do the most basic of tasks.

Self-Regulation

The ability to control oneself is one of the elements of

interpersonal skills. Managing emotions, attention, and behavior necessary for a task in a socially acceptable manner may deem challenging to an individual grappling with social skills.

Relationship Management

If left untreated, a social skills deficit may lead to difficulties in forging and maintaining long-term relationships. Especially in children, during early childhood development, the ability to form friendships is essential because it makes the child feel accepted, loved, and confident.

Survival

It is the wild west in today's social world. To be able to hold your own is an impressive skill that reassures your confidence and trust in people. For example, if you have anxiety and then your school, or office holds a social event, you may be tempted to sneak away to your comfort zone, but it would be for your benefit to adapt to change by remaining in the social space and giving people a smiling nod at the very least.

Surviving also includes the ability to read and understand social situations. When you remain in this event, you get to observe other people and how they interact with each other, thus learning what is expected of you on the superficial level.

Accountability

If you struggle with social skills, in your perspective, competition may be a strange aspect of human nature. You may very well struggle with failure, as well. You may not know how to handle situations if they do not go according to your meticulous plan. With training and practice, you are taught that failure is a necessary step to success, and there is no need to get bent-out-of-shape.

Anger Problems

Without training, social skills deficit may pave the way for considerably greater problems like anger. Because we are social beings, people may anger us and that anger, when expressed negatively, may harm the people we love most. People focus on anger as a prime emotion because it is likely to be more harmful than other emotions; therefore, training on how to correctly channel it would lead to healthier relationships.

Psychological Issues

Stress, depression, and anxiety are prevalent in people who have trouble interacting in society. The psychological torture may sometimes lead to suicidal ideation. Because they are not able to interact with society, they may feel unwanted and alone- self-hate is a powerful emotion that burns like wildfire if unchecked.

So, individuals who have communication methods that cultivate less association with others are bound to wind up depressed. Now and again, this is only the aftereffect of character; however, in different cases, it very well may be impacted by the environment in which somebody has been raised. It is very conceivable this can make somebody progressively helpless against discouragement. On the other hand, when somebody is depressed, it frequently changes how they associate with others.

Drug and Substance Abuse

When people who have been subjected to psychological trauma have had enough, they may turn to unproductive ways to reduce their stress and feeling of loneliness by abusing drugs.

Isolation

The typical way of dealing with stress for a large portion of us is to diminish the pressure and tension by staying away from the distressing circumstances. For other people, avoidance of social situations leads to indulgence in solitude and solitary activities and behaviors, which are difficult to change as time goes by.

The individuals who need to improve their social abilities should concentrate on mirroring wonderful demeanors and taking out bothersome practices. They can utilize demonstrating, acting, and execution criticism to recover their particular social abilities shortfall.

Chapter 4: What It Means to Lack Social Skills

Poor social skills are one of the significant problems that individuals face in contemporary society. It is vital to understand that other than the typical social growth that individuals have; the interaction is a critical element that can only be observed whenever an individual has appropriate social skills. Interestingly, in the universal society, a high number of individuals still don't understand what it means to lack social skills. This chapter will, therefore, address what it means to lack social skills by discussing poor social skills and how it affects human health.

Poor social skills are critical since they not only inhibit an individual from interacting with their colleagues but also promote mental issues. Poor social skills, in most cases, are observed within the school environment, especially among teens and adolescents. It is thus your role to ensure that you are well conversant with the signs of poor social skills to avoid any complexity or future mental issues. Importantly, understanding what poor social skills are also essential since it will make you learn how to socialize with individuals in different environments without any difficulty.

Types of Poor Social Skills

There are numerous types and categories of poor social skills. Poor social skills are likely to be caused by various factors, mainly due to a lack of knowledge, among others. Knowledge wise, poor social skills are likely to be associated with the inability to acquire new skills through interactions. An individual may know how to socialize, but in the real sense, their capabilities to learn may still be poor. Poor social skills may also be caused by both external and internal factors, and thus, it is your role to limit such factors. There are various types of poor social skills, including inappropriate basic communication, poor empathy and rapport skills, poor interpersonal skills, imperfect problem-solving process, lack of accountability.

Inappropriate Basic Communication Skills

Poor basic communication skills are one of the immediate types of poor social skills associated with most of the individuals since it leads to various complexities, which further inhibits a smooth socialization process. Poor basic communication skills are composed of the inability of an individual to listen and follow instructions that are provided by other parties. It is essential to understand that for an individual to interact smoothly and share ideas, they must adhere to various guidelines that are equipped with other parties.

Poor listening skills are, thus, portrayed through multiple means, including failure to nod the head and poor concentration. For you to claim that you are being engaged in a talk, you must be able to follow each move that the speaker gives. Such steps can only be seen through accurate listening and concentration. Therefore, basic communication involves giving continuous feedback on any issue which has been addressed by another party, of which failure to do so clearly shows poor essential communication skills, which is an immediate example of poor social skills.

Failure to refer to various past events and discussions is also an example of poor essential communication since to determine that an individual was keen during discussions or not, they opt to refer to the past. Therefore, to ensure that you adversely resolve the problem of basic communication skills and avoid any complexity, you should stick to eye contact, have a genuine emotional attentiveness as well as physical stillness. It is essential to understand that one of the immediate types of poor social skills is a lack of practical communication skills, which every individual must resolve.

Poor Empathy and Rapport Skills

Empathy and rapport skills are fundamental social skills that every individual must adhere to, and failure to take part in such cases would eventually lead to the poor engagement process. Poor empathy and rapport skills are also contributed by various factors, including mental health conditions and also behavioral issues. However, it is also essential to note that poor rapport and empathy skills are also dependent on an individual's ignorance and negligence. In most cases, people try to assume that rapport skills are mainly required during the interview process, which, in the real sense, is a wrong assumption.

It is appropriate to have a good rapport in any social environment since it not only ensures an individual takes part in the interaction process but also limits special issues such as shamefulness and disrespect. There are some cases identified to be the core reasons for poor rapport and empathy skills, including autism and social impairments. Whenever you notice that you suffer from such disorders, it is thus your critical role to incorporate appropriate empathy and rapport skills in every activity which you engage in, including both informal and formal interaction processes.

Individuals with stipulated social disorders, including autism, are prone to poor interaction since they are limited to little empathy towards one another. To resolve such issues, it is thus recommendable that you take part in displaying appropriate self-consciousness and also limiting various aspects of social anxieties. Such recommendation is therefore suitable since individuals with multiple elements of social anxieties tend to be desperate and ensure that they are engaged in all scenarios to please others. Such individuals are also known to paying too much attention to what other individuals talk about and thus end up being confronted. To avoid such cases, it is, therefore, your responsibility to be overwhelmed in every social environment and also avoid paying too much attention to any individual.

Poor Interpersonal Skills

Poor interpersonal skills are not only a problem in the engagement process but also limit an individual towards learning from others. Poor interpersonal skills are composed of the inability of individuals to share and join other activities. In most cases, it is also essential to understand that such individuals with interpersonal issues tend to complicate every single move that they take. They also have specific problems, especially those associated with failure to ask questions whenever they don't get something clearly. Interpersonal skills are also critical since they enable an individual to build appropriate social relationships without any form of difficulty as they suffer from the fear of exposure.

Due to the failure to ask questions, it is crucial to note that such individuals tend to be demotivated since they follow the wrong directions. Failure to ask essential and vital questions thus leads to numerous problems and also creates barriers between individuals. Whenever such barriers are created, the interaction process is, therefore, limited. Additionally, individuals whose interpersonal skills expose them to failure in interaction thus are seen as antisocial. However, the same individuals with poor social skills are also known to ask closed questions to avoid them from giving individual responses whenever the need arises.

In typical cases, closed questions are known to lack various responses, thus lower the rate of engagement among individuals. In such cases, it is, therefore, the critical role of those with poor interpersonal skills to clearly adhere to open questions and also avoid limiting themselves to specific questions, including nonresponsive questions. As an individual, to boost your interpersonal skills, it is also your responsibility to withdraw any barrier and directly engage others in the interaction process.

Poor Problem-Solving Process

Problem-solving skills are essential skills in every social environment. In every social context, it is crucial to understand that problem solving is a vital tool that ensures that there are limited or no issues which are portrayed during socialization. Problem-solving skills are also vital since it helps an individual in the determination of various problems which and their solutions. Through such skills, it also becomes easy to identify multiple strategies of interaction, and also, an individual is limited in every decision that is made. Limitation in the decision made is a fundamental aspect since it ensures that an individual does not cause various problems to their colleagues, among others.

However, it is also essential to understand that other than determining the root cause of the problem, such skills also assist in ensuring that individuals refrain from making various decisions that are likely to affect or annoy their colleagues in any way. Whenever you are in good terms with the colleagues, it becomes easy to share important ideas that build you both socially and economically. It is thus your essential role to ensure that you do not engage in any activity in which you do not know how to resolve any problem that is related to it such activity. In other words, an individual should make a decision of which themselves rely on, for instance, whenever you decide to interact with other people be ready to resolve any problem. Other than solving various issues during the interaction, it is recommendable to avoid any problem since they eventually lead to an individual being uncomfortable. It is thus essential to understand poor problem-solving skills is an immediate example of poor social ability since it directly leads to the weak interaction.

Lack of Accountability

Lack of accountability is also an example of poor social skills as every interaction or social environment is influenced by the extent of accountability. It is essential to understand that in the conventional society, there is nobody who would wish to interact with an individual who is not accountable since there are some activities which, whenever they are not addressed in terms of accountability, they are likely to lead to many complexities in the future. In most cases, people do confuse reliability and accountability and reliability. Reliability is the process where an individual can be responsible any time without any excuse or issues. Accountability, in this case, refers to being responsible for any blame and any action, whether bad or good. Individuals with such characteristics are those who are termed to be sociable since they can be reached anytime there is an issue that has risen.

Therefore, to resolve such poor social skills, it is your essential role to ensure that you are accountable all the time, and under no circumstance do you take part in any action which is likely to affect your accountability. The stipulated types of poor social skills must thus be addressed to ensure that there is an efficient and interactive social environment.

Effects of Poor Social Skills on An Individual Health

Poor social skills are critical since they profoundly affect an individual in various ways. Such poor skills slowly have an impact on individual mental health, which eventually affects the physical health of an individual. It is essential to understand that most of the poor social skills discussed above are directly influenced by to what extent an individual can think or not. To ensure that an individual think in the right direction and avoid various issues with others, they must have appropriate social skills. Your interaction with others must thus be oriented towards one's mental and physical health.

The stipulated poor social skills are likely to affect mental and physical health since they lead to more stress and loneliness. Since individuals with poor social skills tend to lack a sociable environment with which they can learn and prosper based on their colleagues, they tend to suffer from intense stress. Intense stress eventually has numerous effects on an individual's mental health, which further causes specific diseases such as stroke. Therefore, one crucial way to avoid stroke is by ensuring that you have appropriate social skills such as accountability and good problem-solving skills.

Importantly, poor social skills are also likely to affect the physical health of an individual through physical damages such as involvement in the fight, among other aspects. One of the most evident skills that lead to such instances involves poor problem-solving skills. An individual with poor problem-solving skills tends to cause chaos whenever they interact with other colleagues who eventually lead to a harsh social environment. Therefore, in general, to improve your social skills, you should ensure that you have good problem-solving skills, you are accountable and also master basic communication skills. Adhering to such skills will not only ensure that you have a smooth social environment but also improve your mental and physical health.

Chapter 5: Making Conversation

Are you aware of how to have a conversation? It is not just a boring conversation, but it should be a fantastic, unforgettable, and unbelievable communication. When you are aware of how to begin, then you can have a conversation smoothly as one of the vital skills you can be gifted with — the most requested topic at the science of people in the art of sparkling conversation. There is a good and evil conversation. Bad conversations have a specific sequence of events that will lead to an awkward moment. For example, you can hear statements like "most of the night was awkward and not helpful; thus, I didn't have any connections."

There are situations where you wish to talk to strangers and want them to warm you up. You should put in mind the people around you that will the best in you anytime you speak to them. People you are comfortable to talk to them about, they can be your old friends or a new friend you just bumped into, but the conversation between is flowing. If you can make a conversation that people around you admire, then you don't have to despair. You can learn how to have a meaningful discussion, and this will happen when you have a focus, and your practice to make it better. When going to meet new friends, the biggest challenge you can face is the awkward silence.

Keeping Your Conversation Going

This situation is always an uncomfortable feeling that you may end up avoiding meeting new people in your life. There is a solution to such occurrences. Previously you can find yourself thinking it can't be solved, but when you learn about it, then you can get a solution. When you are unable to keep a conversation flowing, then this can be harmful to social life. If you are aware of how to keep a conversation flowing, then you will be able to meet, talk to anyone, and be reading to know anyone you like. Some ways can help you keep a conversation going, and this will make you have good interactions and make them awesome conversations.

1. **Make the conversation about the other person and not you**

   I am sure you have met people who will talk to you about things that you are not interested in at all. This made you feel like they are having conversations with themselves, and you just happened to be present. Such kinds of people will always be oblivious to the opinion that you may want to share their interests. A good conversation will start with showing interest to the other person, their environment, and what they are interested in. A lot of individuals will always want to talk about themselves, and this is something most of you love. You should ask open-ended queries about things you notice about them. When you give sincere compliments or positive feedbacks, this can be a great start to your conversation. As a great conversationalist, you should have a sincere interest to other people, try to find out anything about them, and the things you get to know about them use them to begin and fuel their conversations.

2. **Learn active listening**

   A lot of people are always in thoughts on what to say next while the other person is talking. You should be cautious about this, and anytime you find your mind going for a response, then stop and, make yourself to be attentive. This is usually difficult when you are extremely talkative. You can learn this by being with your partner or friend and try to do it repeatedly by saying to them what they have said. This process can assist you in bringing a consciousness of the quantity of time you can devote attentively listening to other people.

3. Bring the conversation to deeper levels

Have in mind the people who you are willing to be open with, and you can share your ideas with them. You should be able to tell what makes you feel so comfortable to them that you can easily disclose things to them that you can't tell any other person. This can be due to eye contact maintenance on you, thus making you feel like they have given you full and undivided consideration. You should put into consideration their expressions. You will realize that they are not just with you in their toning of words but also expressions. Their faces will always be bright when you are sharing anything good to them, and they will be excited and feel happy. When you are sharing something bad, they will have a sad face. This will make you feel how much they are engrossed in what you are trying to communicate to them. You may find yourself trying to copy what they have done to you, and it may look difficult to you; thus, you need to practice. You must notice the different reactions from people too.

4. Ask good and relevant questions

You can lure people into sharing more and having an interest in the conversation when you ask open-ended queries that can assist them to be in the conversation. You can ask good questions like asking someone how they feel and think about the issue they are talking about. In cases where you have talked to a person previously, then you can ask them about the things they have volunteered during the conversation previously. They can bring up some topics on their own, and this may be of interest to them and some importance too. You should try to explore more about the related interests that they can be comfortable to talk about.

5. Put into consideration time and space

You should never begin an interaction beyond exchanging fast pleasantries unless you are attentive to listen to the person. If you are in a place where there is a lot of noise with so many people around, then that is not a good place to engage in good conversation. A great conversation needs a slow, relaxed pace and pressure zero atmospheres where are no distractions. One of the best places in the coffee shop. Sports bars cannot be that efficient for good conversations.

6. No clarifying

This is where you are allowed to say anything that is going on in your mind. You should not clarify or check on yourself. You can practice this well without any difficulties by trying it out with the people you know. This can be fun when you realize you are free to say whatever that is in your mind and that no one is going to judge you for what you say. Anything you say is okay as long as it doesn't bring you any problem. Others won't care so much about what you are saying; this is because they will be busy trying to focus on how they are going through.

7. **Try to find more when it's interesting**

It will work 99% most of the time. This is a surefire method, and it's the best for those who are starting. Everyone is always happy when they realize you have an interest in what they are saying, and you are attentive; thus, this will make them hang around and want to talk more to you. When there are a lot of reactionary expressions, then the other individual will be satisfied that you are very attentive to the conversation; thus, they will feel flattered.

8. **Stories from all over**

You are aware that stories will always juice up interactions, but a lot of people will always want to talk about their personal lives. It is not a must that you tell stories from your own experience when having a conversation with someone. You can tell stories from different places, stories that occurred to someone you know, stories about people you met, or read about in the newspapers or listened to via radio. You may be wondering how to incorporate stories into your interactions. The most important thing you first to realize that you can put stories in your conversations. These can be stories that you have heard of and are interesting that you can't forget about them; thus, these are good stories to include in your conversations. Such stories will be impossible to be lost with your mind. When the person you are involved in a conversation brings such related stories then join in despite not being from your life. The story can be silly, short, interesting, or even awkward, but use it.

9. **Act that you are interested**

You can choose topics that other people have a concern and care about. Overall everyone will want to talk about their beings and interests. Your conversation can be rolling when you involve topics like; when you are going to meet someone have topics in mind that can come along in the conversation in case the interaction gets boring. You can ask queries about the person's school progress, their hobbies, their background, and families, or friends. You should always be very attentive as this vital, just like talking, and this will help to enhance the conversation. When you are listening, then you will be advantaged to get to hear the other person's viewpoint.

10. **Give a friendly approach and foe**

You will make a first impression when you meet someone, and this will occur most of the time before you begin speaking. You will think you don't make the first impression until you begin speaking, but this should not be how it happens. You should be aware that before you begin any conversation, you should approach it with a lot of confidence in your body language. At a first meeting, your brain will try to see if the person you are meeting is a friend or a foe.

11. **Bookmarking**

As a talented conversationalist, you should do bookmarking when in a conversation. This is a very enhanced process that you will love, but you have to practice. This is where you have to put extra emphasis on some points in the conversation that can build a great link. Bookmarks are vocal enhancers that will make you have an easier talk. You can mention things about the future that you can follow later. You can also include jokes that rarely happens but are very lovely when they are told. You can find yourself having a similar interest to the other person. You can express how much you are surprised to have a story in common. You can also bookmark with a follow-up indication. You can most of the time talking about books, films, movies, or articles you like to the person you are talking to.

You are now aware of the procedures that can help you make a conversation to move; thus, the next activity to do is to try and enact the procedures with someone. You should not stress and try to employ all the tricks at the same time. You should get one and try to use it before you choose on the others. When you gain confidence in the one procedure that you have taken, then with time, you will be confident to use the other methods too in your conversations. For you to level-up your memorability, then you can practice putting humor in your communications. Try to learn how to be funny despite the feeling that you are not unusual. You can take step by step and be guided on how to be funny so that you can use it appropriately in learning humor. Just keep in mind that you are fascinating, and this will make the other person know that you are dazzling.

Despite the way the conversation goes, the ending should be warm. You should have a new acquaintance despite not having someone to fall for you. When someone is speaking and giving various themes that you can enlarge on. You can take them as great advantages for you to have to improve the conversation.

How to Keep Text Conversation Going?

If you can keep the text conversation moving, then you can be considered attractive or appealing. You are supposed to know how essential to let your fingers talk. Your world should be your playing field from your point of view. A lot of many possibilities for digital communication have been established though so many people still find it hard to match up the longer texting conversations. You can get it so difficult to flirt because of distance. This is because, like many other people, you will find it easy to flirt in front of each other. There are certain methods that you can use to help you master texting for a long time in your conversation.

1. **Give full details**

   Just like fashionable dressing, you must consider the devil is in the details. Any time before you press the send button or key, you have to make sure that the text you are sending is sensible. You can take a second to read your text out loud, and this will quickly tell you whether you should send it. The query should be whether the text you sent can be easily misinterpreted or cold naturally. You should always make sure that it looks right before you allow yourself to send the text. This is an example of where you re-read your exam paper before you hand it over; thus, it's worth your time.

2. **Have an interest in your love curiosity**

   So many people don't want to hear this, but it will be better if you get to know this. You should express interest to the person you are sending texts. A lot of people always do one-way texting; thus, this may be boring, and the conversation may not be appropriate.

You should always give some encouragement to your partner or the person you are talking to always reply with open-ended queries about themselves. The conversation should not be just about you, and you should keep this in mind. You should contact them that you have an interest in what they have to say and what they are thinking.

3. Patience pays

Due to the enhancement of technology, there is no doubt that the current communication works in a very crazy place. This should not hinder you from practicing patience when you want to reply. At times an individual is too busy to reply fast. You should always be cautious before you reply, and you are encouraged to take deep breaths before you reply. You have to enjoy the conversation, and this should be done without any pressure. When you are patient, there will be an attraction you will have for other people, and this can be a great platform for you to practice. For you to look more romantic, end a conversation, and leave the other person hanging where they will want more. Practice won't make you perfect as such, but you will at least be better.

4. Invest in fun conversation

A girl is likely to fall deeply for a guy when there is fun. If you have the masses of interesting things to communicate, then these are the things that ladies will want. You should be friendly, always playful, and calm; thus, this is the right direction. When you always laugh, this can be the best to show to the other person. You should always keep off tension in your text conversations; thus, you will be in the correct move.

5. **No filtering**

When you employ this method, it will allow you to say anything in your brain. This will allow you to avoid checking with yourself before you let anything out. You may doubt yourself most of the time, but when you practice it, then you will get yourself into saying something nothing. You will find it so interesting when you can say anything that positively is in your mind. This will tell that you have confidence in yourself, and you are not afraid to be straight and being honest.

6. **Get to know more when it is interesting**

This can be a good method that works most of the time. When you are starting, then, this can be the best process to use. In human history, everyone will always want to be appreciated and made to feel special. Thus, when you show your partner that you have an interest in what they have texted you, this will give you a step high to get them. When you employ this method, then there is a possibility the other person will open up to you and talk about their more personal data that can the conversation moving on calmly.

7. **Tell common stories**

You are always aware of the stories that will make the conversation to have some interest. A lot of people have been programmed to most of the time talk of their personal stories, but this should not be the case. You should employ stories that both parties have an interest in. You can either use a breaking news story that occurred or some icon story in the papers. You should be able to bring such topics in your text conversations so smoothly. You have to begin by telling the stories, and your partner will give you the feedback. As you communicate, you will realize whether they are into the story or not. When you figure out that they are not interested in your story, then you will be forced to try another topic or story.

The world has evolved with the technology that has been improving daily; thus, this tells you that when you don't get into any relationship, you will keep in mind the master of texting and help make the conversation moving. Always listening to what you are being told, and before you say anything back is patient and calm. After following the methods, you have to understand the patterns of the character you are communicating with to keep the conversation going on smoothly. When you have the skills, then you can always have the best conversations ever. When you employ these methods, then you will see the reason for being in the right conversation. This will not happen within a night, but you need to get some practice; thus, you will enhance your conversation skills.

Chapter 6: Reading Body Language

Body language is non-verbal communication where physical behaviors, instead of words, are used to relay or express the information. Such physical behaviors may include facial expressions, gestures, eye movement, touch, body posture, and the use of space. This non-verbal communication makes up a considerable part of everyday conversations. Experts have suggested that body language accounts for approximately 65 percent of our communication.

Body language can be unconsciously or consciously, and it is vital to pay attention to this body language and non-verbal cues when having a conversation because they convey volumes of messages. Non-verbal communication plays a significant role in conversation in our social interactions, for example, repetition, contradiction, substitution, complementing, and accenting what we say in words. Therefore, it is good to be more sensitive to your body language and those of others to become a better communicator.

The ability to read and understand body language helps you notice the unsaid issues or negative feelings that people may be having. Positively, it can add strength to what you say verbally. Therefore, understanding the use of body language can help you connect better with people, and build stronger relationships, thus, improving your social skills.

For you to understand more about body language, we are going to delve into different body gestures and the information they convey:

Relaxed or uncrossed limbs: Relaxed limbs rarely cross one another, except as a position of comfort. They hang loosely.

- **Arms** - Tense arms are held close to the body and are rigid, but relaxed arms move smoothly or hang loosely. The crossing of arms can indicate there is tension while folded arms may be comfortable.

- **Hands** - During the conversation, and we are anxious, most of the time, we use our hands to hold ourselves or touch ourselves or otherwise show tension. Relaxed hands are used to emphasize what we are saying and hang loosely. Gestures are not tense nor sudden but are generally open.

- **Legs** – Legs may casually be flung out or sit gently on the floor when sitting. Legs can move with music rhythm with tapping toes. They may also be crossed, but not wound around each other. When a person is controlling an upper part of the body and arms, legs can convey a sign of tension. On the table, one may appear relaxed, but the legs may be wrapped and held tense

Open palms: Palms gestures are commonly used in conversations, but do people understand what they are doing or why. There are three palms positions one can form: Closed fist, palms down, and palms up. Each of these forms relays a different attitude during conversations. Therefore, it is essential to master and use them appropriately.

- **Palms down**: Palms down shows dominance, it is used to establish authority and superior attitude. It is a way to tell people you are in control, and you are doing the talking. Intensity depends on how forceful the motion is or how inclined your palm is down. It can also be an excellent way to prevent other people from interrupting your speech. You raise your hand when someone is about to halt, and you ask them to wait, non-verbally.

- Another example is when you raise the hand with your palms towards someone; this way, you are asking for patience. It can also mean you are creating a wall between you and the other person, which is freakishly annoying.

- **Palms up**: When someone comes with palms up, they tell us that they are honest, trustworthy, and have nothing to hide. Our subconscious has accepted this as a credible way to show sincerity. It explains why people who conceal their palms during conversation appear a little suspicious. Also, palms up can signal submissiveness. It is a way to gain trust and support by giving up control. For instance, with your palms up, you ask someone to do something, there is a high chance he or she will accept the request, not as an order but as a request.

- **Pointing**: This gesture can be annoying or useful. When we were growing up, we used it to point at stuff and to learn to count or name. As grownups, we also use it as a tool in teaching. However, pointing at people, especially with the thumb, is rude. It is considered as a sign to ridicule or accuse someone. Therefore, it is best to avoid it unless you are provoking someone.

Pupil size: A lot of time spent having a face-to-face conversation with other people is spent looking at their faces. The signal people send out with their eyes reveal a lot about their attitudes and emotions. The Pupils react unconsciously to stimuli and, therefore, cannot be manipulated or controlled. Your eyes are the means of seeing what is going inside of you. It is why when people meet for the first time, and they make judgments based on what they see.

When an individual holds a gaze, he or she is telling you one of these two things. First, they find you interesting or attractive and secondly feeling hostile or anger. You recognize this by looking at their pupils. In the former case, the pupils are dilated, while in the later have constricted pupils. Pupils will dilate or contract as mood and attitude change from negative to positive and vice versa. When one gets excited, their pupils will get dilated to up to four times the normal size. Conversely, negative moods or anger causes the pupils to contract.

If you are a person who has interests in body language, I am sure you have come across this term before. Negative gestures are body movements that could give a wrong or negative impression on people. Even when an individual does not know how to decode body language, he or she can still manage to get a particular perception of you from your gestures because the subconscious will detect them. Here are some of the postures that are related to negative body language gestures:

Leaning away: Also, it can be referred to as leaning out, which signals people that you are not interested in them, what they have to say, or/and their ideas. This language is pretty much applicable in dating, business, and amongst friends. For example, leaning in when you are on a date with your partner can show her or him that you wish to gain some intimacy, whereas leaning away suggests the opposite.

Also, in a business meeting, when you sit at the edge of your seat and lean in towards a person presenting, shows you are keen to gain information. While with your friends having lunch, when you sit leaning forward as you engage them with a conversation, portray a lot of interest. These gestures all work in reverse to show disinterest.

Crossed limbs: People either knowingly or unknowingly, always read our body language. Crossed limbs have a significant role to play in this non-verbal language.

- **Crossed arms** – Crossed arms can be read by others to mean you are insecure, distant, defensive, anxious, or stubborn.

- **Crossed legs** – It shows dominance and confidence when you sit with your legs crossed, ankle over the knee. It is predominantly male body movement, but it is being used increasingly by women. Ankle lock is crossing your legs at the ankle while seated. It can mean that you are uncertain, holding back, or fearful.

Tight shoulders: It is worthwhile to consider what our shoulders reveal about us. It is not common that shoulders are talked about in non-verbal literature, and the irony of this is that when people are asked about it, they shrug their shoulders. Shoulders are very prominent, they shape what people think of us, reveal our emotions and health, hold up our clothing, and assist us in communicating, and yet still a lot of people ignore them. Although shoulders have limited movements compared to other parts of the body, they can be used to relay various signals.

Shoulders hunched up, usually with arms folded or crossed tight and holding the body, this can be a sign that the person is feeling cold. It can be a sign that the person is in extreme tension, often from fear or anxiety.

When an individual fears attack (actual or virtual), he or she raises shoulders and lowers the head to protect the neck.

Feet turned away: Many people will rarely notice the secret messages their feet are signaling. Our feet and legs reflect our feelings. If a window to your soul is the eyes, then legs must be the signpost to what you are thinking or feeling. People do not pay much attention to how they position their legs when having a conversation than they are with other parts of the body. Therefore, if you are building up your body language, then perhaps it is best you add leg and foot positioning to your cluster of cues.

When you are having a conversation with someone, if his or her feet are pointed towards you, then it is most likely that he/she likes you, interested in what you are saying, and agrees with you. However, if his feet are turned away from you, this can mean that he wants to leave and need to be somewhere else. It almost feels like he is already walking away.

Leaning on two hands or head resting on one hand: You may have noticed people leaning on two hands, or perhaps find yourself doing it and been wondering why. There are some physical reasons as to why you are doing this. Maybe you have been in the same position for a prolonged period, or you are tired, and this serves as a refreshing stretch. But that aside, we want to understand why people are doing this, and what they are unconsciously saying when they assume this body gesture.

The hands behind the head, with a backward lean, can mean two different messages depending on what the hands are doing and where exactly the arms are placed. They are referred to as the cradle and the catapult. Cradle can mean insecurity and a need for comfort, whereas catapult suggests dominance and aggression.

On to the head resting on one hand, is with no doubt revealing our true feelings and thoughts-despite what we say. This posture is telling us that the person is uninterested in the current situation and is a sure sign of boredom.

Neck body language: Neck is used to rotate and support the head, therefore controls some head body language. The neck can also relay few signals of its own.

- **When hiding** – Neck is where a predator will aim, either going to rip out the windpipe or jugular artery at the side. When people feel an imminent threat, they will react to protect the neck. Some people can do this by pulling down the chin to protect the throat, and others may raise their shoulders to defend the sides of the neck.

- **Turning** – The neck can be rotated to enable us to look in many directions. It is useful to extend our range of vision. It can also be used to deliberately send a signal that an individual is removing or giving attention. The neck can also be rotated to exercise it, which can signal tension or indicate boredom.

Shoulders body language: Shoulders too can be used to convey a variety of signals:

- **Raised shoulders** – Raised shoulders and the lowered head is used to protect the neck when the person fears an attack.

- **Curved forward** – This happens when one folds the arms. When shoulders are curved forward and hands down, it reduces the width of the body and, therefore, can be a defensive posture, just a desire not to be seen, when an individual is feeling threatened.

- **Pushed back** – When shoulders are pushed back, it forces the chest out, exposing the torso to potential attack. It shows the person is not afraid of attack, and it demonstrates power.

- **Circling** – This is done backward or forward, with both shoulders or one. It is done to exercise a stiff shoulder, which may have resulted from tension indicating anxiety. It can also signal that the person is preparing themselves for action, perhaps combat, and, therefore, can mean aggression. When done while the other person is talking, not minding to listen carefully, can be a signal of power.

- **Shrug** – Classic shrug is a one-off raising and lowering of shoulders, which usually means "I don't know" and can be done with raised eyebrows. A quick shrug and performed subconsciously may indicate a lack of understanding. It can also mean uncertainty. When a person shrugs instead of speak can signaling to lie as they fear their words may give themselves away. An animated and prolonged shrug can indicate preparing for aggression and thus signaling a threat. It can also indicate frustration or irritation in a smaller form.

- **Turning** – If a person turns their shoulders still looking at you, it probably means they want to leave. Perhaps because what you are saying is beginning to sound uncomfortable for them.

Chest body language: The chest can send some non-verbal body language signals. Some of the signals include:

Thrust out - Thrusting forward your chest draws attention, and can be a provocative romantic display. Women, for example, know that men are aroused when they see breasts. When women push their chest forward, they may be inviting intimacy or just teasing.

Men also push their chest forward to display their strength, except that for men, they do this both for women and other men. In the case of women, the man is saying, "I am strong and can protect you," while for other men, he is suggesting (I am strong and would better not cross me).

Withdrawn – The chest cavity contains very vital organs and is vulnerable in case of attack. When pulled back, it indicates the person is attempting to hide or appear inoffensive.

Leaning – Leaning forward close to the other person can have two meanings. First, it can show interest in the other person. It can also indicate more romantic interest.

Secondly, it can invade the space of the other person, thus posing as a threat. It is aggressive and often shows in dominant body language.

Hips body language: Hips are at the base of the body trunk. And without any doubt, they do signal certain messages in body language. Some of the common body language signs include:

- **Thrust out**: Hips have primary sexual organs, and trusting them out is a provocative and suggestive gesture.

- **Held back**: This is the opposite of thrusting them forward, it hides the genitals, to prevent them from being noticed.

- **Pushed sideways**: This makes the spine curve, and a result rearranges the whole body. It is a relaxed position as an individual lets the body drop. It can also be used as a subtle pointer indicating what the person wants. When pointing at a person can mean they are found to be attractive. Pointing at the exit may mean the person wants to leave.

- **Moving**: Hips moving from side to side is largely a common dance move indicating one may like to dance. It also attracts attention to that part of the body and hence inviting flirtatious actions. Moving hips back and forth, simulating sexual intercourse and can be arousing.

Hands body language: Hands are the richest source of non-verbal language, after the face, of course.

- **Holding** – Cupped hands symbolize holding a fragile idea. It also can be used to give, whereas gripping can indicate ownership, possessiveness, and desire. People can also use their hands to comfort themselves, for example, holding their own hands. Holding self can also be seen as an act of restraint, letting the other person talk. It is used when the person is with anger, to stop them from attacking.

- **Control** – Hands are used to greet people, and the most common way of greeting is shaking. For example, prolonged holding, using more strength, and the other hand, to hold the person can show dominance. Submission is revealed with a floppy hand, the palm facing up, and a quick withdrawal. Most of the handshakes are done with vertical palms, which indicate equality, which lasts for the same time.

- **When asking** - Palms upwards is commonly used as a plea gesture, while palms downwards can mean asking the other person to calm down. Palms pressed together, with fingers upwards- the prayer position- indicates a more anxious pleading.

- **Rubbing** - Rubbing the hands can indicate the person is feeling cold. Massaging hands together is an indicator of anxiety and stress when the hands are tense. Rubbing the chin can signal the person is evaluating, deciding, and thinking.

Leg body language: Our legs can tell a lot without us realizing it. It is because people normally focus on the upper body when they want to control their body language. Legs conflicting with the rest of the body show deliberate control and thus signaling what people are thinking.

- **Open standing** – Standing with feet open about the width of your shoulders is a relaxed pose and normal. A wider stance makes one appear bigger, hence signaling dominance and power.

- **Closed standing** – A person standing with feet put together displays some anxiety.

- **Crossed legs** – Crossed legs while standing can mean shyness, especially when hands are held at the back and lowered head. When sitting crossing legs can take many forms, for example, an ankle cross and tucking your legs under the seat, can show concealed anxiety.

- **Moving** – A crossed leg and be moved up and down, and this can indicate impatience. A leg can also swing to music, meaning the person is enjoying the vibe and is relaxed.

- **Walking** – A person with a fast walk shows he or she is in a hurry, while a slow walk indicates the person has time to kill. However, unaffected walk indicates self-consciousness; the person is concerned with how others perceive them.

Body language in communication is something that one needs to understand as it is key in determining your personal and professional relationship. Being aware of body language can make us understand people better and thus improve our social skills. It is because we can decode the signals they are sending and react accordingly, depending on how we understand them. However, if we do not understand how to read these body gestures, it can be chaotic on how we relate to others. It is, therefore, an important thing to be aware of how other people or we use their body gestures to improve our relationships with them.

Chapter 7: Telling Stories in a Conversation

It doesn't matter the occasion: it could be that exciting family get together or a casual outing with a friend or even a date with your love, being able to tell entertaining stories in your conversation without being boring will help you pass time and impress your listeners.

The skills of good storytelling could mean the difference between getting that dream job not or being in a relationship or not. However, for many people, the skill of storytelling seems out of grasp. You certainly want to do everything to avoid being a boring sour storyteller when you are conversing with others. Being a poor storyteller can be quite discomforting, you will keep looking at your watch wondering when your meeting will end. This could interfere with your listening skills as you pay little or no attention to what the others are saying, well because you don't know how to respond in an exciting way.

What is more, almost all world leaders are avid storytellers. It is one of the critical skills you can pick up. You, therefore, need to be a very good storyteller for people to start listening to you. However, you should note that this skill cannot be learned overnight. You need a lot of time and practice in order to develop your storytelling skills over time.

The following are some of the tips that can turn you into an avid storyteller:

- **Pay attention to the opening of your story**

  You need to pay a lot of attention to the opening part of the story more than any other part. It doesn't matter if you are speaking to a crowd of 1000 people or across your seat with just two listeners. You should aim at grabbing their attention and making them part of the story from the word go. One of the best ways you can do this is by making your story sound real, relevant, and rich. You should also fill your story with specific sights, smells, and emotions that reinforce your theme. Ensure you make your audience feel they are part of your experience.

- **Listen and retell**

You need to think about all the interesting stories told by others and retell them to your audience. These stories are most likely a result of the experiences which others went through in the past. Most of the best and interesting stories are from bad experiences you went through or which others went through. A good story should be about an unexpected event and how you or others reacted to them.

After identifying a story that fits the occasion you need to retell it in the most interesting and captivating way possible. Describe the vents vividly and be careful to add suspense to it. If it is about something you witness or experience you should have a clear picture of what happened, and you can, therefore, recall it with great detail and accuracy.

- **Set the context**

Before you start telling your stories, you should first set the context of your story. You probably have of the details of what happened in a particular situation, but unfortunately, your audience doesn't. You, therefore, need to bring your audience on board by giving them details that answer the questions who, what, why, where, and how. You should do this when you at the beginning just when are introducing your stories.

Setting the context is important to enabling your audience to follow your stories without getting lost or being confused. It also makes them feel they are part of the storytelling; thus, you get and maintain their attention throughout your conversation.

- **Set the mood**

In addition to setting the context, you should also set the mood of your story by setting the tone from which the story takes place. The tone of your story is important in affecting the listening experience of your audience. Avoid speaking in a monotonous boring voice.

Moreover, ensure you make constant eye contact with your audience. Making eye contact helps you to keep your audience engaged and attentive throughout your conversation.

In addition to eye contact, you must also make use of appropriate gestures. Using gestures will help the events in your story flow better and also give life to character s and their actions. Gestures also help in giving a physical sense of momentum to the way you tell your stories.

Another aspect of non-verbal communication cues you can incorporate to make your storytelling exciting and memorable is your voice projection. You should try to vary your tone to bring out the different characters in the story. You can also do this by making use of mimicry. If you can mimic well how a particular charter speaks, you will make your audience be so engrossed and engaged in what you are telling them.

- **Include your emotions**

  Captivating stories are not all about what happened and when. They should reveal how you felt going through a particular experience, how you reacted and what motivated you into finding a solution. These are details that make your audience relate well with your experience. The more emotions you include, the better to make your story as interesting as possible.

  Creating an emotional connection with your audience will keep them engrossed in every word that comes out of your lips.

- **Allow your audience to imagine**

  When you are telling an oral story, you should allow your audience to imagine it. Encourage them to participate in and visualize what you are narrating. You can do this by asking them to guess what happened next before revealing to them. Avoid the close-ended questions which will elicit a simple yes or no answer, instead ask questions that will make them guess what happened.

  You should also avoid describing every detail, instead give them the bits of a scenario and allow them to imagine the rest. For example, you can say," I met Barrack Obama at the cinema, guess what he told me?" they will then imagine the scenario and guess what actually happened after.

- **Make use of casual familiar words**

  Avoid using confusing wordy jargon while narrating your stories to others. Your audience will not only be found some of these jargons quite confusing, but it will also make them lose interest in what you are saying pretty fast.

  When you are telling your stories, make sure you use the lay man's language. If your audience fails to understand what you are saying, then you are wasting your time and theirs too.

  If you are coming from a science background or other related complex field, avoid scientific terms when explaining the latest trends in your career to a crowd of people at a party. Instead, use common language to tell them what is happening and why it is important as well as how it will affect them

- **Include dialogue**

  Ensure you include dialogue in your stories. Dialogue helps your story to come to life. Tell your audience what others said using their own spoken words. For example, then he told me," lie down, or I shoot." I immediately went down, then he asked me," do you have any money? give me your phone."

  Dialogue also helps your audience to live through your experience and get your message clearly. You can also use dialogue at the Climax to tie up several events in the story and make it effective.

- **Avoid giving out unimportant details**

  It is very easy for you to get lost in your own stories,

especially if you choose to give out too much or unimportant details. If your mind tends to wander off when narrating stories, you need to learn how to edit your thoughts so as not to bore your listeners to death. Giving too many details will also get your lost and may not follow well what you are saying.

It doesn't matter how exciting and fascinating your sidebars are, in the end, it will only serve to distract and frustrate your audience. It will also turn you into one of the most boring storytellers whom everyone would want to escape from.

- **Get to know your audience well**

Choose stories that won't offend your listeners. Avoid offensive themes or parts that may make your audience quite uncomfortable in their seats. For example, avoid parts that broadcast your resources in front of an audience who are less fortunate. Such stories will not only make you insensitive in front of your audience but may also make them develop a negative attitude toward you and what you are saying. Ensure you edit such parts or, where possible, delete it completely.

- **Add a few details of your own**

It is often said there is nothing new under the sun, and well, the same applies to stories. If you are retelling a story either from your own experience or stories you heard from others, then you should add a few details of your own to give it a fresh perspective. However, you should be careful about how you do this. Add a few details without spinning the story further away from what happened. The more you drift a story from what exactly happened the more you are tempted to describe events that never happened, and your story will end up sounding far-fetched and untruthful.

- **Rehearse what you are going to say**

It is advisable to run your story through your mind before telling it to your audience. You can easily do this as you drive to your meeting venue or when you are taking your meals. Get to rehearse every detail in order to build up a good plot. You should also plan on how you will present the conflict to your audience in such a manner that will instantly draw them into your story. You should also plan how you intend to end your story in the most captivating way.

A good plot should have the beginning, where you give the audience the context of the story, then followed by a rise in action, this is where you introduce and develop the conflict then followed by the climax of the story and finally resolution.

- **Be considerate of others**

If your story involves other people, be careful not to reveal sensitive information about them. If your friend has trusted you with some of their secrets, be careful not to reveal such information to third parties in the course of your storytelling. For example, you will sound inconsiderate if you reveal the sexual orientation of others whether they are close to you or not. It will also be quite uncomfortable for everyone if the said person is within hearsay.

- **Keep your stories short**

  There is no one as boring as someone who keeps talking for hours nonstop. You should be careful not to bore your audience with long stories. The average attention span of people is quite short, and you must restrict your stories to the appropriate time limit. You should aim at telling stories that will last 2 minutes at most. Anything more than that will quickly turn you into a bore. You are also forcing your audience to put too much attention on you when you draw your stories for too long. Remember, a good storyteller must give a chance to their listeners to speak also. Allow them to interject, ask questions or tell similar stories of their own too.

- **Be attentive to what impact your stories are having on others**

  You should be keen on what impact your stories are having on your listeners by observing their non-verbal cues. Some listeners can become quite preoccupied and disturbed by your stories especially stories s relating to a difficult experience you went through. You should be careful not to repeat too much negative tinged stories during one sitting. You should also prepare your audience well in advance before telling them a sad story. You should also avoid giving too many details of such sad stories or telling them for long as this may end up stressing your listeners.

  Finally, telling stories is one of the natural and enjoyable parts of your social interaction. You should incorporate the above tips to tell stories that will keep your audience attentive, fascinated, and happy.

It is also important to note that your storytelling skills are proportional to your practice. When you strive to engage and stay relevant to what your audience needs to hear, storytelling can become a meaningful experience for you through which you can improve your social skills.

Chapter 8: How to Declutter Your Mind

I know you imagine that there is nothing that could compare to an untidy home and workspace. But I am here to tell you there is, and that is a cluttered mind. I know you are now probably wondering, "a cluttered mind?" "How exactly can a soul be untidy and full of unnecessary stuff?" Well, according to experts, a cluttered mind is one that is full of negative thoughts, keeps on worrying about things way out of their control, and is holding on to past hurt, anger, and resentment. Also, the same mind is easily distracted and has persistent sensory input.

A cluttered mind is easily distracted, is confused, and has problems making decisions. It wastes not only your time and energy but also distracts you from what is essential in your life. It makes you lose touch with yourself, the present, the environment, and those around you. A cluttered mind focuses on many things at once, and as a result, very little gets accomplished. It makes you disorganized and unproductive in your day to day activities.

The good news is, there is a solution to your cluttered mind. You do not need to move around anymore, like a robot with minimal performance. It is time you let go of those toxic behaviors that you have become accustomed to, and that is preventing you from attaining your full potential. However, you will need to set your mind to it and be intentional about what you want to achieve. It will require you to choose wisely where you spend your time and energy and what exactly your attention will be focused on. Then and only then will you slowly move away from those unhealthy thinking habits that have given you a mind block and are limiting your potential.

Below are some of the ways through which one can de-clutter their mind and gain focus:

1. **Ensure you get adequate sleep**

    Research has shown numerous benefits of sleep to your physical and mental wellbeing. These include improved memory, better moods, improved immune function, and a healthier heart. Lack of adequate sleep is linked to higher incidences of heart diseases, depression, and cancer. Therefore, it is evident the benefits sleep offers to your mental health. Inadequate sleep will leave you tired, irritable, and less productive throughout the day. You will experience a brain fog throughout the day that will interfere with not only your interactions with people but also how you carry yourself and make decisions. Researchers have gone ahead to explain the effect of inadequate sleep on your brain cells. It interferes with how brain cells communicate with each other interfering with your memory. Thus, you will experience temporary memory lapses throughout the day, interfering with your productivity. If you are having difficulties falling or staying asleep, you should consult a health care provider for professional help. Either way, ensure you get at least six hours of sleep every day. Do not let inadequate sleep get in the form of your day.

2. **Get time and meditate**

    In the modern world, life has become so hectic that it is rare you find time for yourself. Take, for example, a working mother. She has to ensure she prepares her husband and children before they leave in the morning before she can make herself and go. At the office, she has deadlines to meet and demands from the boss that a matter of time and death. Let's not forget that she has her son's graduation to attend, her daughter's game to visit, and parents meeting at the end of school. She then has to come home to prepare food and put her children to bed before she can clean the house and then herself retire to bed. It is all within her typical day of 24 hours, and the cycle continues. Such a woman rarely has time for herself.

But here is the thing, no matter how hectic it is, always set aside time and meditate. You could join the local yoga class that happens in the evening after work, or you could take your lunch break at work to sit by yourself and meditate. Meditation goes a long way in helping you de-clutter your mind. It makes your mind to a place of clarity and reason. It helps clear out the fog that is keeping you stuck and limiting your potential. It helps reduce the confusion you are facing by helping you see the clear-cut lines that have been drawn in decisions that have to be made. It helps take your mind away from what is distracting you and focus all your energy and attention on what is essential. With all these benefits of meditation, it is clear you need to make meditation your daily routine.

3. **Write down your thoughts**

One thing you will need to appreciate is that you are human, with a human brain and memory. You are not a computer somewhere that is capable of processing millions of data at a go while storing millions of others. When you understand this, you will appreciate the power of writing down. Not just writing down the responsibilities you have to accomplish by the end of the day, but also your thoughts, dreams, and ambitions. Get yourself a haven for yourself, either in the form of a physical journal or digitally on some online blog. With time you will realize the positive impact writing is having on your life.

For one, writing relieves you of the responsibility to remember what you have to do throughout the day. It goes a long away in helping de-clutter your mind. Besides, if you are the creative kind who is always generating ideas, writing provides you with a way to channel your thoughts and assess their viability. It also helps create some headspace for more views and goes a long way in helping de-clutter your mind. If you are trying to solve a problem at work or home, writing down your options will go a long way in helping you get a clear picture of the situation and make a decision. Writing also helps calm the many voices in your head that are causing confusion, creating peace for you, and de-cluttering your mind. According to research carried out by the University of Rochester Medical Center, journaling was proven to be a crucial tool in helping manage mental health.

It is evident writing has so many benefits to your mental health. Therefore, ensure you try to journal every day. Make it a habit even when you do not have a topic to write. With time it will become more comfortable and you will find yourself writing more every day.

4. Set priorities

Being an adult is not easy. And no one promised you it is going to be easy. There is so much to be done in such little time. You end up feeling overwhelmed and de-energized to carry out your responsibilities. Each day make sure you make a list of what is expected of you by the end of the day. However, minor it might seem, it needs to be done by the end of the day, so ensure you jolt it down. Then take time to categorize all the day's responsibilities into urgent, important, and non-important. The urgent issues must be completed by the end day; otherwise, there will be severe unintended consequences. Something somewhere will go wrong if you do not accomplish urgent matters. It is the equivalent of someone dying if not achieved by the end of the day. The important responsibilities need to be completed, but no one will disappear if it is not accomplished. The non-important matters require your attention, but life can go on if they are not attended to.

When you organize your day's activities this way, you will be able to know which one to attend to first and which one should not worry you. You will have a clear picture of how your day is going to proceed. Whom you are going to meet and what you will discuss. Who will be left pending until later in the week, and who needs to be called? It helps clear your brain of the fog that was crowding your mind. You will be able to make well-informed decisions. You will be so energized for the day that you will surprise even you. With each goal that is accomplished, cross it off your list so you can know what you have done and what is yet to be done.

5. Organize your working space

With busy, hectic lives, comes untidiness and disorganization. Your desk will be full of papers that need to have been cleared like last week. You will have a laundry basket full of dirty clothes yet to be washed, a sink full of dirty utensils. In short, everything in your life needs to have been done like yesterday. Untidiness creates chaos both in your life and mind. Research has shown that an untidy environment occupies part of your brain. It restricts your thinking and creates a brain fog. It is because the chaos is continually competing for your attention with your tasks at hand.

You cannot relax at home or your office because of the chaos around you, and you cannot think clearly or make decisions because of the untidiness around you. The only practical solution you have is clearing out what needs to be removed and cleaning the rest. Organize your desk and home. Ensure everything is tidy and is where it needs to be. This way, your brain will be able to process information efficiently helping you make sound decisions. You will be focused on whatever task is at hand. Your energy levels will go up improving your productivity.

6. Avoid multi-tasking

Some of you are mangers at one or more companies. On top of that, you have your personal life to take. You have a social experience to attend to and friends to appease. These are a whole lot of activities for one person to perform at a go. You may be tempted to carry out several tasks at once, or otherwise known as multitasking. You are at home cooking dinner, and at the same time, you are writing the report for the week's activities. Also, you are supervising your son as they do homework, and you are on call with your boss at the office. When you are performing several tasks at once, your mind is not set on one thing. Instead, it is thinned out on all the activities you are playing. It clogs your brain and reduces your productivity and ability to make sound decisions. You will end up not accomplishing much at the end of it all. Besides, you are as tired as a log with little to prove why you are as tired. Instead of multitasking, organize your activities into urgent, important, and non-important. Set your priorities right. Carry out each task at its own time to protect you from a mental overload. If you are so pressed on time, you could get yourself a timer and set time for how long you want to carry out each task. It helps you manage your time effectively.

7. **Enjoy nature**

You are so busy such that the only environment you appreciate is that of your home, office, and the journey in between the two. What you do not know is that the world has so much to offer besides those clumsy environments that you have now become accustomed to. There are so many beautiful sceneries for you to appreciate, but you are so pre-occupied with work even to notice. There a beautiful waterfall that is your way to work, but you have never visited it. You live next to the beach, but the number of times you have visited the beach is countable. Most people do not appreciate what nature has to offer. It is free, yet you would rather spend thousands of dollars talking to a psychiatrist. I am not saying it is wrong. It is just that we underestimate the power of taking that walk to the edge of the forest behind your house. Or going to the beach with the family on an afternoon. Studies have shown that being in nature has several health benefits including decreasing anxiety and depression. It helps trigger your mental status while restoring it to normal functioning. Nature helps improve your moods and boost your energy levels thus increasing your productivity. Therefore, the next time you felt down and overwhelmed, take a stroll, go swimming, or go running in the woods.

8. Limit your internet time

Let's appreciate that we live in a technological world where the internet is freely accessible. There is a lot of information that is easily accessible over the internet. Be it on social media, blogs, or online magazines. Being always on the internet impacts your life in different ways. It provides too much information to your brain, more that it can handle. It ends up clogging your mind reducing clarity and productiveness. It also adds on brain clutter and even harms your mental health creating loneliness, thus increasing the risk of depression. Therefore, you must limit the amount of time you spend on the net and even go ahead to define what kind of information gets to you. Though we cannot disregard how important the internet is in our lives, you must filter the information you get into what is essential and what is not.

9. Exercise

When is the last time you were at the gym exercising? Okay let's not go there then, when is the last time you ran on that treadmill that is in your house? I am pretty sure the answer is a few months or even years back. Exercise has become such a foreign term in the modern world, that it is slowly losing its meaning. Yet, extensive research has been done on the benefits of exercise to the body. These include losing weight, regulating cholesterol and sugar levels, and a healthy heart. What many don't tell you is that exercise is good for the brain too. It helps the brain release endorphins, which are known to improve mood and memory. Thus, exercise helps unclog your mind and keeps you on your toes helping you make sound decisions. It sharpens your memory and decreases the risk of developing depression and anxiety disorders. Therefore, before you skip your next gym appointment, be sure of the benefits you deny your body.

Mental clutter clogs your brain and prevents you from seeing things clearly. It reduces your productivity and leaves you feeling tired despite being unproductive. But the good news is that you can de-clutter your brain to help yourself perform better. To help yourself live the best life you ever have so far despite the day to day challenges that you face.

Chapter 9: How to Develop Your Mind

Developing your mind relates to the physiological memory where the mind trains the functions to your body in other words, if you do not change ways in how you do things then your mind will not be at work because it is already used to whatever you are doing but if you are forced to do it differently it activates your brain and its functions. Your mental development does not only end in school, but it is also applicable in the outside world. That is why mental life is all about interest, while physical life is all about happiness, remember to keep that in mind. There are several ways to develop your mind, and they include:

1. **Read the right type of books**

    Reading enables you to learn new things about people and places. It also stimulates your brain through imaginations and improves your understanding in different ways by preparing you for new opportunities.

2. **Learn to think creatively**

    Do not underestimate yourself for things you cannot do instead of thinking of the things you can do and apply your thoughts and ideas in your life as it challenges and engages your mind. Do not stop thinking creatively until your ideas and thoughts push you to a new ground.

3. **Exercise regularly**

    Daily exercise is healthy for your physical health and mental health. Many people tend to think that exercising only helps physical health; however, in mental health, it reduces stress, triggers your memory, attention, and ability to move quickly between different tasks.

4. Meditate

Meditation practices improve your mental function; that is how you make your decision and how you process information as well as your moods and your well-being as a person.

5. Learn new skills

You should learn new skills such as engaging in playing games, learning new languages, and trying new activities and hobbies because they force your mind to work and enhance your mental functions.

6. Cultivate curiosity

Learn to question things even if they seem to be necessary or obvious; maybe you want to know why a sure thing is how it is and why it works in a certain way don't just accept things the way they are. You also need to explore by visiting new places, eating fresh foods, dressing differently, attending different and unique ceremonies because this makes your mind build new connections anytime it meets something difficult to understand.

7. Diet

There are certain foods you are advised to eat that can

improve your mental function, concentration ability and protecting your brain from degeneration such foods are foods rich in omega-three like fish, foods rich in magnesium, antioxidant-rich foods like fruits and vegetables and foods rich in the whole grain like brown rice.

8. Taking short notes

Writing down brief information while listening to someone during a meeting, class, or conferences helps you to recall what was said and to integrate it thoroughly.

9. Focus and review

You should focus on learning about the new ideas that you come across anytime as it improves your thinking, then you need to revisit and rehearse the new concepts learned because it helps you to memorize it quickly.

10. Avoid smoking

You should avoid smoking and using illegal drugs at all costs because it reduces your level of memory and planning, as well as your mental ability overall.

11. Get enough sleep

Sleep is essential as you are always advised to sleep for 8hrs a day as it improves your mental function, helps in your concentration, and keeps you alert every time. Sleep also prevents the loss of gray matter in your brain.

12. **Involve your senses**

Involve your five senses to help you try and relate to new information given to help you understand and recall it. You need to know different tastes, feelings, how they smell or images as it helps you to remember something effectively.

13. **Brain games and puzzles**

There are several online games in your phones, laptops, or computers that are challenging for you to solve this helps you to expand your thinking skills, activate, and keep your mind engaged.

How Antisocial Can Improve their Social Skills

If you are an antisocial person, a shy person, or a person who feels awkward and nervous at any social event and gatherings like family events and public places, this can affect your social life and career. If you improve all these that have been mentioned above, it can help in your social life. That is how you interact with your colleagues at your workplace and how you relate with others outside. Here are some ways that you need to follow to improve your social skills:

1. **Read books about social skills**

Reading certain books can help you learn precise social skills and remember to practice them repeatedly, for they help you to start conversations with different people that you meet with. If you only read books about social skills and not put them into practice, it will not help you in any way.

2. **Practice moral behavior**

   You need to practice excellent communication skills like being polite when talking to someone older or younger than you, use words like excuse me and please when you need something and remember to know how someone is feeling or has woken up by greeting them. Practicing moral behavior goes hand in hand with improving your social skills.

3. **Identify and replace negative thoughts**

   Always believe in yourself that you can start a conversation with someone, meet with new people, and end the discussion in the right way. Don't have the mind that if you start a conversation with someone, you might embarrass yourself and make yourself feel bad because this may lead to no one not recognizing your presence in an event and when you leave, you to start blaming yourself that you are an awkward person. Identify the negative thoughts that are not productive and are dragging you down then replace them with realistic thoughts.

4. **Behave like a social person**

   I know this might be difficult for some people, but it will get easier as time goes by, and it will help you improve your social skills. Start conversations with new people and involve yourself in discussions with other people for you to know something. Don't let your anxiety hold you back.

5. **Encourage others to talk about themselves**

   Ask others about themselves like what they like doing, their careers, family, and how they have been then showing interest while listening to what they are saying. You can also start to tell them about themselves and your experiences to make the conversation going. Most people like talking about themselves.

6. **Offer compliments generously**

   Compliments are also ways that start conversations with someone. You can begin by complimenting how smartly dressed your colleague is at work or even the presentation your employer made at a staff meeting or something new your friend bought like a new car or a new laptop because compliments show how friendly you are.

7. **Ask questions**

   You can get people's attention by asking open-ended questions in a meeting. Ask questions that do not require a yes or no answer as it enables other people to gain interest in knowing what you want to know, and this opens conversations. Encourage other people also to talk.

8. **Make goals for yourself**

   Make goals that can help you improve your social life as if you want to practice a specific social skill or if you want to join a social activity like visiting orphanages and providing the orphans with the basic needs they need like food and clothes. For you to communicate better, you need to learn and use the smart goal.

9. **Start small talks**

   Going to public events and spending time with new people may seem complicated, so for you to get used to it, you can start short conversations with the shopkeepers in the stores by saying thank you or greeting them first before saying what you need. Practicing small conversations often improves social skills.

10. **Stay up to date on current events**

    Visit social media most of the time, find what is currently trending and new stories about celebrities or what is happening in the country so that you can have something interesting to talk about with people and avoid politics because some people are not a fan. This can be a great way to start conversations.

11. **Body language**

    You should always know that nonverbal communication is essential, so maintain eye contact, stay relaxed and keenly listen to what the other person is saying to give you the idea of what to say next whether you want to answer a question, ask a question, or make a comment. This also opens the door to conversations.

12. **Join social skills support groups**

    You need to join at least the support groups for they enable every member of the group to say something about themselves and people in the group get interested they ask you questions, and you answer.

This will make you start practicing social skills and will result in you making conversations with people without being shy and afraid.

Techniques Used to Master Your Social Skills

Learning social skills can only be done with the help of other people you are close to, like your friends, siblings, parents, and teachers. Patience is the only virtue that you need to have for you to master the skills because no one is born perfect, and it takes effort to nurture the skills. Here are some techniques that will help you learn your skills:

1. **Stories**

   You are always told stories by your parents, teachers, or even friends, and at the end of the story, you need to have learned a lesson or two when you were listening keenly. Stories guide to improving your social skills, and from what you learned, it would enable you to master social skills.

2. **Games**

   Several challenging games need problem-solving. The purposes of these games are to interact with others and improve your social skills. These games not only improve your social skills but also enhances your communication skills from reading, writing, and speaking.

3. **Practice**

When you don't put your skills into practice, they will never improve because practice makes perfect. The daily conversations that you have with people have much added to your social skills because it is part of practicing. If you put your expertise in use today, then tomorrow it will give you the chance to practice it.

4. **Using their names**

Using other people's names in a conversation will make them become interested and put a smile on their faces than using your name in a conversation. You can make more friends by being interested in them other than making people interested in you.

5. **Eye contact**

Maintaining eye contact can be disturbing to some people; however, it increases friendliness and attraction. If you keep an eye, contact it will bring your concentration close to what the other person is saying, thus mastering the social skills being used.

6. **Smile**

This leads to happiness and friendliness between the two people conversing during a conversation. The smile makes it difficult for someone to like you, and you will be surprised to know that everyone likes you and would like to communicate with you. There is a social skill that comes with a smile.

7. **Vary your tone**

   When you vary your tone during a conversation, it will possibly keep other people want to engage and get interested in you and what you are talking about. The charming people always use the tone; that's why people like them.

8. **Innovative questions**

   These are the type of items to be used during a boring conversation. You should ask questions like "what do you like doing during your free time?" ask them what they wanted to be in the future when they were kids, show them that you are interested to know more about them. These questions will make one involved in a conversation.

Chapter 10: Changing Your Social Behavior

You may have some awkward feeling that you are poor when it comes to social events, and this may make you have so many struggles to be in conversations. This can have some impact on your social lifestyle and occupation. When you have great social skills, this can be vital to help you in impacting good friendships and having a great life in the outside world. When you see yourself as an introvert, then you mind finding it difficult to get into communication with the people you are not aware of or similar to. The more time you take to practice, the easier you will have to feel.

How to Change Your Social Behavior?

1. **You should act like a social person**

   You are advised to try and act like a social being. Just force yourself even if you can't do it. You should never allow yourself to be pulled back by stress. You should always make decisions about talking to the new people that you meet to get into conversations even though you are feeling nervous. As time goes by, you will get it easy, and you will improve faster; thus, this will help to enhance your social skills.

2. **Begin small if forced to**

   If you are going out for a party or you will be spending your time in a crowd, and this looks overwhelming to you, then you can begin small. When you get into a grocery store and say thank you to the person that offered the services to you, then this shall prove how you are practicing; thus, the small talk will grow gradually.

3. Ask open-ended queries

In cases where you wanted to be given undivided attention or be listened to, then you have to be asking the other person open-ended questions. You should cheer the other person to talk to avoid the conversation being idle. The questions that you ask the other person should require more than a yes or no answer, and with this, the other person can always keep the conversation going calmly.

4. Cheer the other person to talk about themselves

A lot of people will possibly feel good when they talk about themselves. When you ask someone about their occupation, what they like, their families or friends, this can make them feel close and open to the conversation. You should always express your interest to the stories the other person is telling you. The conversation you are having is upon you to make it go, and you can do this by including games like ping pong.

5. Enhance your personal goals

You should try to set some small objectives or goals for yourself. You can decide to begin practicing some particular skills, or you either begin to attend some social operations in your society. You should try and find a goal and begin to work on its approaches that will help to enhance your social lifestyle.

6. **Give generous compliments**

   When you have compliments in a conversation, then this can be a direct way to have a good interaction with the other person. When a co-worker is presenting something, then try to compliment it, or when you see your neighbor or friend with something, always give a compliment. For instance, buying a new car. When you compliment, then this is a sign of being friendly, and the other person may be generous about your compliments.

7. **Go through the book, articles that are associated with social skills**

   When you visit libraries or the market, you will come across so many books that can assist you in developing specific social skills and different methods for you to begin conversations. You should always keep in mind that the reading you do about social skills will not make you a genius. After reading the books, you are supposed to practice the skills most of the time for you to master them.

8. **Have a good character**

   When you have a good character, then this will go in hand with enhancing your social skills. You should try being polite, show gratitude to the other person, and maintain good table manners.

9. **Listen to your body language**

   Non-verbal interaction is very vital. You should always be attentive to the kind of body language you are using.

You should look relaxed, try to make the right amount of eye contact, and try to be free and open to the conversation. Teach yourself to know how to practice your physique language appropriately.

10. Engage yourself with social skill care groups

A lot of societies will give social skill care groups. These kinds of groups will be there to assist you and the other shy person, feels awkward, or is tremendously nervous when it comes to social situations and to practice the new services. You can begin to improve your social skills; thus, this can fuel you to make new friends that will be there to comprehend your difficult moments or situations.

11. Be updated on the current issues

You should always be updated about the current news or trending issues so that you can always have an idea or something to share with the other person. Avoid controversial matters that will be of no interest to the other person like politics. The stories you talk about should be of interest to both you and the other person. This is the best way for you to begin a conversation and help you maintain neutral themes.

12. Get to know the negative thoughts and replace them

When you are full of negative thoughts in your mind about your social interactions, then this could tell that it has become a fulfilling personal insight. For instance, you may think you are awkward and can embarrass yourself and end up being alone at some corner at a party. This may make you leave the party earlier than expected with thoughts that you are awkward because you talked to no one. You should get to know the negative things that are pulling you down. Try to replace them with some real impacts, and for example, you should be able to tell yourself that you can make a new conversation, and you can meet new beings. You should never entertain the thoughts that are not any products to be inside you.

13. **Have a visual program**

A good way to help challenge character is by making it very simple for kids to try and foretell what will be ahead or next in their plan. For you to assist in this situation, then you have to make a simple and something to read for the kids with the help of words and pictures to show various events and happenings. You should always go through the plan daily with the kids and the whole class, plus those who will require some extra assistance with the transition. You should have a good design of your plan to help in removing items as you cover them.

Importance of Communication Skills

Communication skill is very vital when it comes to the creation of friendships and the building of a robust social support system. It also assists you to be careful of your wants as you also become respectful to the desires of the other person. No one is always born with excellent communication skills like the other skills, but these skills are learned through practices where you will have to try and fail, and this is a process to be repeated severally. There are three parts of interaction that you will possibly want to be aware of:

- Non-verbal communication

- Assertiveness

- Conversation skills

You should put into consideration that there are several aspects to excellent communication, and you may feel like you need some assistance in particular areas. For example, you may want to know how to solve conflicts, how to present something to people, how to give feedback, among many other things.

Non-Verbal Communication/Interaction

A lot of communication that happens between you and the other person is non-verbal. The things that you will tell someone with your eyes or body language will be as effective as the words you will tell someone. When you are nervous, you can be in moods that will make you not want to talk to anyone around you. For example, you can end up avoiding eye contact with other people, and in cases where you speak, it will be very soft. In short, you will be not ready to communicate. This can be because you don't want to be judged negatively by people.

Nevertheless, the body language that you portray and the tone in your voice will be able to tell others about your emotional state, your attitude to those listening, your knowledge about the topic, and your level of honesty. So, it may be possible that when you avoid eye contact, be some distance away from people, speak softly, then this means that you don't want to be with your friends. People may come up with an assumption that this was not the message you were to send.

Conversation Skills

A big challenge that you can experience when you are a nervous person is how to begin a conversation and keep them moving. You should know that it is very reasonable to try small talks because it may not be easy to bring into discussions about what you have in mind. This can be true when you are anxious. In other cases, some nervous people may be talkative; thus, this can create some negative imprint on other people.

Assertiveness

This is one of the most honest expressions of an individual's wants and feelings, and it will have respect for those of other people. Communicating assertively will enhance your manner, thus being non-threatening and non-judgmental. This will make you take responsibility for your actions. In cases where you are socially nervous, you may find it very difficult to express your thoughts and feelings openly. Learning may be complicated, and this is because you have to hold yourself back from the things you used to do frequently. For example, you fear conflict, going out to crowds, and fear of giving your opinions or suggestions. This may bring about the development of a passive communication style.

You can choose a substitute to control and take over others and try to enhance a hostile communication style. The assertive interaction style will bring about several aids. This can make you communicate with other people comfortably, without any anxiety and bitterness. It also gives other people the benefit of living their own good lives. There have been so many myths about assertiveness. Some people claim that it is a method that you get your way all the time. This is a lie because being assertive is a way of expressing what you think, and you communicate honestly with other people.

Other people think that being assertive is being mean or selfish. This is a false phrase, and because you are expressing your opinions, that does not mean that you have forced other people to believe what you are saying. When you express yourself assertively, then this will be an advantage to the others as you will have given room for them also to speak. You can be assertive to someone else. People feel that when you are passive, then you will be able to agree with others. This is a wrong statement.

When you are inactive, then you will approve with the other people; thus, this will allow them to be on their paths. This can help them to have their wishes, have no demands to request on their own. When you behave in such a manner, then there is no guarantee that other people will have some admiration for you. This may make them see you as dull, and you may be frustrated, causing others not to know you. Excellent social capabilities are significant for you to have a good interaction. When you get yourself in situations where you find interacting with others to be a challenge, then you have to practice the suggestions that have been talked about and try to practice them effectively.

Chapter 11: Manage Shyness and Social Anxiety

Shyness is a sensation you feel whenever you are uncomfortable or awkward when you meet new people or get exposed to unacquainted situations. Shyness can really affect your life and career choices because you are not in a position to talk confidently with the people you meet in every aspect of your life whether at the workplace or home and social anxiety happens when someone has excess fear to face a public place.

Symptoms of Social Anxiety

People with social anxiety always think that they can get embarrassed or judged with other people anytime they talk about something which may lead to humiliation. They tend to avoid social situations and crowded places like interviews, group conversations, and parties. You should know that social anxiety can lead to total isolation. You can understand that you have social anxiety if you experience the following symptoms anytime you face a crowded place or when you are told to make a public speech:

- Blushing in that you avoid eye contact and tend to face down anytime, you want to talk

- Shaking

- Sweating

- The mind goes blank, and you lack the strength to communicate

- You have the urge to use the washrooms

- When you want to escape and leave the place, you are

- Vomiting

- Dizziness. You might even fall down

- Stomach upset at times

- Heart palpitations

- Difficulty in concentration

There are several behavioral symptoms that someone suffering from social anxiety may also tend to have because of their fears, and they include:

- Always avoiding eye contact

- Focusing on yourself and coping with the safety behaviors

- Leaving an event prematurely without talking to other people and telling them where you are going

- Avoiding social situations like parties and public places

- Always keeping quiet during conversations, staying with your ideas from people because you fear to get embarrassed and judged

- Trying not to draw attention to yourself

- Still sitting alone and isolating yourself from others

- Avoiding the situation altogether

Causes of Social Anxiety

People tend to confuse social anxiety with shyness or depression; hence, social anxiety is not always recognized. It is one of the most common mental problems leading to a chronic disorder that may cause impairment over time and vary in levels of severity. Some complications have been identified to cause social anxiety, and they include:

1. **Low self-esteem**

   If a person tends to avoid social places and new people with the fear of getting embarrassed or judged with what others think, it may take a lot of time to improve their social anxiety. Social anxiety for a long time may lower a person's self-esteem leading to social isolation.

2. **Alcohol problems**

   Consumption of too much alcohol is one of the main issues that people with social anxiety have, and they tend to rely on alcohol to help them with their social situations; however, alcohol is a problem itself. Alcohol abuse leads to some chronic disorders that may need you to talk with a health expert about your alcohol consumption.

3. **Depression**

   Depression is a disorder where a person feels he or she has no hope for the future, low mood, feeling that they don't matter, and worthless and loss of appetite and sleep. People with social anxiety often suffer from depression, which may lead to someone having thoughts of committing suicide. If you have experienced the above symptoms, especially the idea of committing suicide, you are advised to visit a therapist who can give you drugs to lower your depression.

4. **Benzodiazepine dependence**

   It is prescribed for social anxiety and other anxiety disorders. They are so addictive, and you can have the withdrawal symptoms if you stop using the drugs; however, they are not treatment of choice.

Genetic and environmental factors also add to cause social anxiety and to treat your social anxiety, you need to know what is maintaining the problem and not focusing on why you have the problem. Slow breathing in that you breathe using your lower stomach and not your chest muscles is also one of the ways that help to cope with your social anxiety, you are advised to relax your stomach as much as possible and only breathe through your nose. If you put this to practice, you will see change.

Treating of Social Anxiety and Shyness

People with social anxiety are also encouraged to learn some informal and interpersonal skills to help them overcome their fears. There is also a specific therapy known as cognitive behavior therapy, which is a treatment of choice for social anxiety. It is all about changing the way you think, feel, and behave in social situations. This therapy can be offered either face to face or through the internet. The treatment includes:

- Being educated about social anxiety that is attached to each person's needs.

- Ongoing assessments about a person's level of social anxiety

- Training in strategies such as training someone to be aware of the social anxiety symptoms and how to manage the anxiety symptoms. You are also encouraged to put these techniques into practice regularly if you need help.

- Mental involvements. You should be in a position to monitor your thoughts and know your thinking misrepresentations during specific situations during the day. This therapy enables people with social anxiety to recognize and challenge their fears.

- Behavioral involvements. This is where the treatment focuses on an individual feared situation. It is when a person is afraid to talk to people in a crowd, but they would like to, they are encouraged to start by involving themselves in small talks with those they are close to, and if they put this to practice they could be in a position to gain confidence and talk to the public with confidence.

- The therapy also helps people who think they embarrass themselves and get judged in society anytime they talk. It gives them the courage to be able to confront their uncomfortable situations by increasing their power of exposure.

- People with social anxiety are also encouraged to identify and let go of their safety behaviors like avoiding eye contact with those who are engaged in a conversation, always being isolated and sitting alone, and speaking in low voices that someone cannot hear. They believe they cannot do without their safety behaviors.

Everyone tends to get nervous during social situations like interviews, crowded rooms, during big presentations at work, and while meeting new people. However, some people are just naturally anti-social than others. When you always have constant fear and anxiety about something, you should visit a health expert because you might have a mental disorder. There are sure signs you need to watch if you are dealing with this mental disorder because shyness and social anxiety may have similar symptoms. At times social anxiety is mistaken to be shyness.

Types of Social Anxiety

Social anxiety disorders can affect both your physical and mental life as it requires treatment to manage this health issue. Once you start worrying about embarrassing yourself in front of people, having anxiety before facing people, being fearful in public, avoiding social gatherings, sweating, trembling, feeling tense, dizziness, nausea and avoiding different situations what so ever are some of the frequent symptoms that you are suffering from a social anxiety disorder. There are two types of social anxiety disorder:

1. **Social interaction anxiety**

   This is whereby someone is afraid of talking in front of a crowd or talking to new people with the fear of getting embarrassed or judged if they try to engage in a conversation because they are not used to engaging in conversations.

2. **Social performance anxiety**

   This is the fear of someone engaging in social activities such as parties, family events, and sporting events because of meeting new people who they are fear talking to. They tend to avoid eye contact with people because they lack confidence; hence, they keep their ideas and opinions to themselves. Both disorders are brought about by the fear of getting embarrassed or humiliated in front of people.

Here are some of the signs to show that your shyness is a social anxiety disorder according to the mental health experts:

1. **Your anxiety seems unwarranted**

   This is when you believe something negative will happen during a social gathering, even if you have had positive experiences in the past. This occurs when you have the fear or doubt of talking with other people that you are not used to, the new people you meet with at the social events. You keep thinking that those people are unreasonable and unwarranted, making you not to trust them. This often makes you keep your ideas and opinions to yourself and not wanting to engage in other people's conversations.

2. **You avoid social events altogether**

   Social anxiety disorders start when you start avoiding social situations, crowds, gatherings, events, and public places altogether. It's not bad for someone to have some alone time, but if you begin to be alone continually and skipping the social events because of fear and anxiety, visiting a health expert could help you know why you are always afraid and anxious. When you get the treatment, it will be possible for you to manage the social anxiety disorder, if you start noticing excessive worry, socializing with people leads to distress or fear of facing a crowd of new faces it is time to consider your shyness as social anxiety.

3. **You are scared of participating in a social event.**

   We all know that shy people always avoid crowded places or social gatherings because they might be told to talk to the public, which makes them feel drained. However, if it gets to the point that you are always worried about getting embarrassed or judged or being fearful about a social situation, this means that you could be having a social anxiety disorder.

4. **You have an overall fear of social situations**

   This happens when you start getting nervous of certain social situations to avoid the fear of social situations you can start by trying something new like visiting new places and attending parties just to meet new people and make new friends or even starting small talks like making a speech and telling stories to those who you are close to. If you practice all these, it will make you overcome your fear. However, if you experience fear of facing social situations, it is a clear indication of social anxiety disorder.

5. **Your relationships are negatively affected**

   Being antisocial can make it difficult for you to make new friends, this making it hurt the links you have with your friends and family. However, having a social anxiety disorder can make you feel impossible at all to make new friends. It is said that once a person starts to experience difficulties in their relationships that were once comfortable, it is a sign that your shyness is a social anxiety disorder.

6. **You are overly anxious about getting embarrassed**

Nobody likes to embarrass and humiliate themselves in front of a crowd however when it becomes too much that you can't even try to talk in front of a group because of anxiety and distress it can be an indication that you have a social anxiety disorder and you need extra support from a mental expert.

7. **You experience physical symptoms**

If you are nervous during a social situation, it may lead to feeling butterflies in your stomach, and you might be having a social anxiety disorder. You experience sweating, rapid breathing, trembling, nausea, and dizziness whenever you may be having anxiety or distress. You are advised to visit a physician for treatment.

Overcoming Shyness and Social Anxiety

Studies have shown that the number of adults who suffer from social anxiety and shyness has increased. However, several effective ways can help you overcome your shyness and social anxiety, and they include:

1. **Be mindful**

Don't get lost in your thoughts; be aware of your feelings, thoughts, memories, and sensations at any time. If you are always present at any moment, you will realize that social interactions are not something that you need to avoid. You should participate better in paying attention to the conversations you are having with others in a particular environment, and this will give you ideas to know what you are supposed to say with those you are conversing with. When you keep this into practice, it will improve your social skills and make you feel more confident. Being mindful is simply being aware of something.

2. Body language

Maintain eye contact with those you are having conversations with. Your voice should be clear enough for everyone to hear and walk with your head held high. This will show the others that you are confident, and no sign of social anxiety and shyness will be shown, making others be interested more in what you are saying. Shaking hands and hugging people is also a way of showing friendliness and closure between you and those who are involved in the conversation.

3. Engage

Engage in small talks with new people you meet at parties, stores, and sporting events. Ask people questions about themselves, ask them about their experiences in life and careers you can also tell them about yourself to keep the conversation going. If you meet someone who you are attracted to romantically, don't be shy to ask them out for dates or even a dance. Take chances for you to meet new people, life is too short.

4. **Act confidently**

   Be confident in a way that you engage in conversations, ask open-ended questions during meetings, and talking positively to someone by making eye contact. Confidence is all about actions, learning, practice, and mastery. Take, for example, if you learn about new things, it is always terrifying at first, but after you have gone through it and tried it, you feel confident. Social confidence also works in the same way. If you eliminate avoiding things in your life like avoiding conversations, you will overcome anxiety.

5. **Make yourself vulnerable**

   Many people tend to get embarrassed or being judged anytime they make conversations with new people, and this contributes to social anxiety and shyness. To overcome this fear, you need to make yourself vulnerable. Making yourself vulnerable is showing people the real you, be proud of who you are. Practice this by engaging in social activities with those you are close with, and you trust this will make you feel closer to others. Being vulnerable and genuine about yourself are the qualities people will appreciate about you and like you.

6. **Try new things**

   Try new things like joining different clubs, attending parties to meet new people, visiting new places, attending various religious ceremonies, and eating fresh foods even if they make you nervous. Just do something new to keep you out of your comfort zone, by practicing new activities it helps you overcome shyness and social anxiety and developing confidence in several areas in your life not letting fear or humiliation get into your way. It also makes you learn how to handle that anxiety more effectively.

7. Talk

Social anxiety and shyness are not reasons to stay quiet. Confident people always talk and not bothering if others are going to like what they are talking about; they speak their minds to share, connect, and engage with others. Whether you are at your workplace or with your friends, practice talking openly, let your opinions and voice be heard. Be more talkative and expressive in all areas of your life. Start practicing by giving speeches, telling stories, and jokes at every opportunity you get.

Chapter 12: How to Improve Your Social Skills

We have discussed that human beings are social creatures, and good relationships are crucial for the physical and mental health of an individual. Poor social skills or social awkwardness can be improved through training and practice. The most important thing to remember, however, is that building social skills is about trial-and-error. You may succeed in one strategy with one person, and the same approach may fail with another. This is because you are dealing with different people and dynamics; it is not just about you. Allow that failure to motivate you to try again with a third person, and so on.

Smart social skills are also known as social intelligence or "street smarts," and they measure how well a person can interact with others. Social intelligence can be acquired, and it has its advantages. Why is it essential to improve social skills?

Therapeutic treatment to assist with social abilities challenges is critical to:

- Help connect fittingly with others during play, discussion, and in communications.

- Help create companionships at school, office, and extracurricular activities, for example, playing sports, going to a gathering, etc.

- Help you to carry on properly during associations with commonplace individuals, for example, guardians, kin, instructors, family companions, and new people such as grown-ups and youngsters they may need to draw in with during journeys and when visiting places, for example, the recreation center.

- Help in building up your consciousness of social standards and to ace explicit social aptitudes, for example, reasoning, alternating in a discussion, maintaining eye to eye connection, understanding figurative language.

- Create suitable social stories to help show you how to react in specific social circumstances.

- A few people require unequivocal instructing about how to connect and speak with others as these abilities do not fall into place easily for them.

The following are some of the commonplace tips on how to improve your social skills:

1. **Study and behave like social people.**

   Most aspects of socializing have more to do with attitudes and thought patterns. Observe social people, how they feel, conduct themselves, and their overall presence in a room. Then go out and practice these skills. Do not allow anxiety to hold you back, learn by apprenticeship. Do not shy away from fumbling over your thought process or words on your first try; it gets better with practice.

2. **Make friends with friendly people.**

   Remember that you are the average of the five people with whom you spend most of your time. Therefore, when you surround yourself with friendly people, you will learn these skills by affiliation; and the more you learn, the easier it will be for you to practice because you have seen your friends do it efficiently. These people may also challenge you to immerse yourself in social situations to sharpen your acuity, which will build your confidence.

3. **Start small.**

If fully immersive social situations are too nerve-wracking, you can start by saying hello to strangers as you take a walk. There is a man I once knew who had a high-achieving strain of autism. To improve his social skills, he went into a fast-food restaurant every day and ordered the same meal- so that he could speak to the attendants and make an order. That short conversation of which order of fries to get, with what toppings, and drink, meant a lot to this man. Yet, he did it every day.

4. **Pay attention**

The mere act of giving someone your full attention without necessarily saying much is a necessary step to improving interpersonal skills. Active listening makes people trust you better, and so they are inclined to share more with you. With time, you may decide to let them in when you are ready. Gradually, your relationships will begin to improve, one-by-one. Focus on other people's interests; you will gain more friendships this way because all your attention is on them.

5. **Understand yourself**

Before you understand the social environment, you must evaluate yourself first. How do you respond to social events? Do you like it when people say hello to you? How friendly do you feel? When you understand which areas you are lacking, you will know precisely how to address your deficits. Understanding yourself will help you recognize similar emotions in other people.

Building social competence is not about changing who you are; it is about improving on that person. Most people are opposed to developing these skills because they feel forced to integrate with society. However, when you understand yourself, you get to see that acquiring social skills only adds to your character not take anything away. You can still socialize in a way that aligns with your values, morals, and personality.

6. **Improve your basic communication skills**

Effective communication skills are at the heart of any smart social skills. It begins with verbal fluency and the ability to express yourself appropriately. Non-verbal communication is just as significant a part of effective communication skills. Learn from observing the people around you. Sometimes people give you social cues, and you must pay attention to see them.

Pay attention to your body language as well. Try to appear relaxed, calm, and confident in your social interactions. Engage your body the right amount, and employ eye contact as wisely as possible. Start with an upright posture and eye contact when you meet someone; your handshake should be firm and yet not overpowering.

Understanding communication skills help you understand conversation etiquette. When you start small, the next step would be to carry the conversation until it dies a natural death. However, do not pressure yourself to engage even when the conversation has gotten away from you; it is okay to move on- either by walking away or sparking a new topic. Active listening will help you with this.

7. Compliment more

Compliments are a good opener, "Nice shoes," for example. Then the other party carries the conversation forward either by talking about shoes or opening themselves up to you for the direction you want to drive it. Compliments show that you are a friendly person, thus paving the way for meaningful relationships. As you learn to give more compliments, also learn how to take them. Most people do not know how to take compliments and end up making a weird situation out of a genuinely good thing.

8. Ask open-ended questions

When talking to someone, ask questions in a way that allows them some answering leeway. Open questions offer a lot of insight into a person's train of thought. When you allow people to talk about themselves, they will go on and on. This is good for you- at least the beginning. Encourage them to share more of themselves with you and listen attentively to ask more follow-up questions.

9. **Learn about conflict resolution**

How do you respond to conflict? Do you fight or flee? Are there people in your life who can offer you honest feedback on this? The ability to solve disputes is vital because conflict is bound to brew in a social setting.

10. **Read more books**

Read more books to improve basic reading and comprehension skills. Reading helps expand your vocabulary as well as improve your thought processes. Not only that but reading more on social skills may help you understand yourself better and how you relate with other people. Reading can also help you with the ability to follow the author's thoughts and increase your visualization skills.

11. **Role-play**

Imagine different scenarios where you are about to engage people. Think of the things you would say to get their attention first, then maintain it. For example, you meet colleagues for cocktails at happy hour. What do you say? "May I join you?" or "Is this seat taken?" And if perhaps you have disagreed with a friend you were having lunch with, "I think we are spinning out, tell me again why you think humanity is innately evil, and I will tell you my opinion after," maybe the appropriate thing to say. Create all these scenarios and more in your imagination and have fun with the different responses and why each is either appropriate or not.

12. **Join a support group**

Many people like you feel overwhelmed in social situations. Finding a supportive group of friends who understand your daily struggles may help you amass confidence to do it all over again the next day. The best thing about support groups is that some people have made it through worse situations and survived to tell the funny story- in retrospect. In a support group, you will be in very experienced hands to guide you through overcoming social skills deficits.

13. **Supplant negative thought**

Replace all negative thoughts with positive. Negative thinking merely does its part to make you feel worse about yourself; it drags you further into the pit of despair. "I will probably stand at the corner of the room at the party" or "No one will notice me at the meeting" or "I would rather go home and sleep than drive in the rain for a family function that only asks about my relationship status." All these are examples of all the negative thoughts we feed ourselves without cause or prompt. They are examples of how much dislike, and how little trust we have for ourselves. Replace all the negative talk with a positive thought, "I will talk to two different people tonight at the party," or "I will ask a question during the meeting," and so on.

Negativity holds you back from your genuine potential, you are destined for greatness, but all the negative self-talk keeps you from achieving it. Most importantly, if you speak to someone with a negative attitude, and you cannot replace the negative with positive thoughts, you are allowed to protect your energy by ending the conversation and walking away, if possible.

14. **Set a goal**

Things may appear to move significantly faster or much slower in a social event, so having a goal is the best way to make the most of it. Set a goal to talk to at least two people in a gathering, or ask questions in a meeting, or plan some productive outcome for your presence in a social event. Establishing a goal will help you devise strategies to achieve them and improve your social skills.

15. **Practice, practice, practice**

Figuring out how to interact with individuals is one of those wide aptitudes where the practice is especially significant. Having some harsh rules as the main priority consistently makes a difference. Also, on an increasingly all-encompassing, backhanded level, you will have a simpler time talking with people if you are an intriguing, educated, composed individual. Being more composed and open to conversations with acquaintances all begin with a single courageous step. Practice good manners, table manners, conversation etiquette, and appropriate body language, and so on. With time, all that seemed hard at the beginning starts to occur naturally.

16. **Be assertive**

At first, it may seem uncomfortable expressing what you genuinely feel if you are used to conceding to others. However, with time, assertiveness feels more natural, and you can relate to others in a way that meets everyone's needs. It is okay to say "no" if the situation calls for it, and it is also crucial to ask for exactly what you want. Assertiveness reduces anxiety and helps you interact comfortably with your peers.

17. Show empathy

Building empathy as a skill is the cornerstone of social interactions. People like to feel heard; therefore, when you empathize with them, they will draw closer to you.

18. Manage your relationships

Striking up a conversation is easy enough. So now everyone at the office knows your name. Then what? Managing relationships is the hard part of all social interactions. You will need to invest yourself in the relationships you consider valuable. Learn to be patient with people and learn how to manage your expectations and theirs. However, keep an open mind and adaptive mentality to the ever-changing dynamics.

19. Complete training courses

There are programs instructed by professionals where they train you on how to improve social skills by evaluating you, then using that assessment to construct activities tailored for your deficient areas, and then give feedback on improvement. These courses are necessary for people who would like to shed the anxiety and social fear. They help model your behavior into practical communication skills.

20. **Become an ambassador**

Pick up a leadership role in whichever sphere of life you are in now. It takes a conscious effort to improve on a skill. Therefore, placing yourself in situations that demand you to rise above your comfort-zone will work to better your social skills and improve your health.

Becoming an ambassador means that more people will talk to you, you will have more responsibilities, you will be accountable to someone for something, etc. This sort of exposure will push you out of your shell and into the arms of society who are willing to embrace you- but do not let them smother you with their insatiable needs. Here, you will also learn how to manage expectations, failure, competition, and so on.

21. **Boost your confidence**

Do whatever make you feel most confident; for most people, it is grooming. When you have worn your best, look your best, feel your best, you are simultaneously more confident. For other people, it is a support system; some people feel more confident when they have someone supporting them in their lives. For other people, achievement gives them that boost of courage. Being confident assures you of emerging on the other side; victorious or not, you will survive to fight another day. So, do whatever you need to do to face your social fear with newly found confidence.

22. **Be active**

Involve yourself in social circles and conversations, whether locally or online. Do not give "I don't know" as an answer to anything; give it a guess instead. Do not avoid uncomfortable situations; face them head-on. Understand what is required of you and buckle down. Even when the last thing you want is to be in a social space, involve yourself anyway.

23. Smile

Some irritable people take social interaction very seriously. It is not wrong to focus- once in a while- on the goofy side of socializing. Smiling makes you look approachable and friendly. When you smile more often, you invite people to feel at ease when they are around you. The smile should be natural, not forced. Forced smiles do not have the same effect as they appear harsh and insincere.

24. Remember names

Train yourself to remember names at the drop of a hat. People like to hear their names being called out; it is like sweet nectar to a bee. Remembering names shows people that they made an impression on you and that you value them.

Social Skills Training

This is a type of cognitive-behavioral therapy that may be conducted either in a group format or individually to improve social skills in people with developmental disabilities or mental conditions. SST has proven effective in teaching how to manage social skills deficits better. Preparation is necessary on the doctor's end because the patient may be dealing with a disorder that may require special attention and specific treatments.

The technique starts with the therapist asking you a series of questions to determine which social situations you grapple with the most. The goal of this exercise is to determine which areas of skills to target during SST. Once the fields are identified, a training technique is introduced, usually tackling one area at a time to avoid overwhelming the patient. Then, the therapist may describe a specific situation and ask the patient to explain it in fine detail and model the behavior. For example, how to introduce yourself, the patient is asked to go into the nitty-gritty of self-introduction, "Stretch out my hand, raise my gaze to make eye contact, shake hands firmly yet not too strong, and say hello, my name is John." Afterward, the therapists give feedback on the performance and talks about body language and non-verbal cues.

SST can be adjusted to the treatment of depression with attention to communication skills, in particular, assertiveness training. For example, depressed patients regularly benefit from:

- Figuring out how as far as possible to other people,

- Getting fulfillment for their very own needs, and

- Feeling increasingly self-assured in social collaborations.

Research recommends SST for patients who are depressed because they are prone to isolate themselves from others can profit by figuring out how to expand positive social cooperation with others as opposed to pulling back.

SST might be utilized to show individuals explicit arrangements of social capabilities. A typical focal point of SST projects is relational abilities. Another primary focal point of the SST project includes improving a patient's capacity to see and follow up on expressive gestures.

Treatment of factors that cause a deficiency in social skills should not involve one therapy treatment because one technique treats one particular shortcoming. Therefore, SST only tackles one aspect of social skills, and overlooking the rest would be an act of negligence. The issues will keep cropping up until they are well addressed and curtailed. Homework and follow-ups are useful in producing long-term results. A study demonstrated that a group that received follow up check-ups showed remarkably more improvement than the group that did not.

One of the challenges facing SST is perhaps the transferability of skills from the doctor's office to the "real world." For example, people with developmental abilities to be able to practice their newly acquired skills more effectively. Future research should also explore the integration of different cultural spheres, mental disorders, etc.

SST is useful as part of a more comprehensive treatment comprised of multiple components, for example, SST is used with other therapies to treat social anxiety by managing the social skills deficit, and the anxiety. Building and enhancing your social aptitudes is a significant part of treatment for social deficit disorders and is essential to better social circumstances. If you end up seriously inadequate with regards to social skills, chat with your medical practitioner about training or different techniques for improving your capacities.

Conclusion

Thanks for making it through to the end of *Improve Your Social Skills*. Let's hope that you loved the content and that it was informative in addressing matters of communication and human interaction. The book is aimed at equipping you with the social skills that can help you improve your interaction processes including general communication, holding conversations, small talks, big talks, and addressing social anxiety and shyness.

The next step, in this case, is to initiate the life itself by recalling each social skill of holding successful conversations and maintaining long-term social relationships. Let's also hope that you will recall the step by step process to address heated arguments as well as how to get along with just anyone. Most of your invaluable time can be spent on helping you ensure that you reach out to friends and potential influential networks that will improve your social, emotional, and professional wellbeing.

Studies have shown that social anxiety and shyness are normal occurrences that most of us face when holding conversations, especially before a group of people. That is why we have comprehensively covered the right strategies to address these issues in order to enhance your confidence and self-esteem while presenting before others.

Finally, if you found this book useful in any way, a review on Amazon is always appreciated!

Self Esteem Workbook

Discover the practical strategies to start believing in yourself and boost your self-confidence and mindset for living your life to the fullest.

Jack Gilman

Introduction

Self-esteem is one of those things that is often talked about by psychologists and clients across the globe. What exactly is the meaning of it? It is a term that is used very often but people don't really know it's the true meaning. The dictionary states that the definition of self-esteem is "confidence in one's own worth or abilities". Many people also use self-esteem interchangeably with self-worth and self-respect. In layman's terms, self-esteem is a crucial part of defining someone's success. However, don't think that having loads of self-esteem will mean that you can achieve success faster. The truth is, that you need to have a healthy and balanced level of self-esteem for it to produce effective results for an individual. Often, people who have low levels of self-esteem tend to fall into depression or self-destructive behavior. It may lead these people into making bad decisions or end up in unhealthy relationships. On the other hand, having too high levels of self-esteem can lead to narcissism. That's not great either! In this book, we will be exploring in detail the different ranges of self-esteem and help you identify where you are on the spectrum.

So why is self-esteem such a talked about subject in the present day? Why is there an almost 10-billion-dollar industry just dedicated to self-help for those suffering from low self-esteem? The simple answer is our fast-paced society. The world we live in present-day moves so quickly and is obsessed with the usage of social media, making it very easy for everyone to compare themselves to others. Most people are guilty of actively following celebrities on Instagram to gawk at their wealth, success, and good looks. In today's world, we are constantly exposed to the top 1% and with the help of social media, we can take a detailed look into their extravagant lifestyles. Being able to see this incredible, yet rare, success makes it difficult for many people to see their own self-worth which then leads to low self-esteem.

Although the constant comparison we are making of ourselves and the top 1% is detrimental to our self-esteem, our upbringing and childhood also play a large role in affecting our level of self-esteem in the present day. If an individual grew up in a strict family who never gave position recognition to them, or they were always overshadowed by another sibling or if they grew up with uninvolved parents and they were always left to fend for themselves, then this will affect their self-esteem later on. Scientific studies have proven that children who grew up in families that didn't show them enough love typically showcased lower self-esteem compared to children that grew up in families that expressed more love.

These aspects are the reason why self-esteem is extremely important today. In the present day, people must always remind themselves of the things they have achieved no matter how significant or insignificant they think it is. People must actively and continuously work on their self-esteem and other similar factors in order to achieve a healthy life. Self-esteem is the biggest influencer when it comes to the important act of decision making. Self-esteem also functions as a motivational tool by making it more or less likely that people will care for themselves to reach their full potential. Self-esteem is definitely an abstract concept because of how difficult it is for those that have low self-esteem to understanding what it's like to have a healthy self-esteem. It is the same the other way around where those with healthy self-esteem find it hard to understand what it feels like to have low self-esteem.

If you are still having trouble determining if you have low self-esteem or just trouble understanding the concept, I will provide you with a few examples to explain further. For instance, imagine someone who really enjoys riding their motorbike. Motorbiking is very important to them so they will take good care of their motorbike and make sure it is properly maintained. They will make good decisions regarding where to park their motorbike, how often they get it serviced, and how they ride their motorbike. They may even build their own custom motorbike and share their passion with other riders with lots of pride. Self-esteem is just like that, except in place of the motorbike, it is yourself. As we mentioned above, children who grew up believing that they were important and valued by their families grow up to properly take care of themselves. In turn, they make better decisions for their lives in the future to enhance their own value rather than diminishing it.

So now you may be wondering, will improving my self-esteem change me as a person overall? The short answer is yes. Just like the motorbike example, by improving self-esteem, you will be helping yourself make better decisions with your life and feel happy in your own skin. By having a healthy level of self-esteem, you will begin to see changes in not only yourself but will affect external parts of your life such as family, friends, and relationships. When you have healthy levels of self-esteem it will eventually bloom into increased self-confidence. Self-confidence is crucial in career development and improving relationships with people in your life.

Throughout this book, I will be focused on teaching you the fundamentals of self-esteem, self-confidence, self-awareness, and self-acceptance. At the end of this book, you will be able to understand the differences between all those aspects and how you can work towards improving all of them. You will be taught the long term and short-term benefits of having increased self-esteem and confidence. I will guide you through a 10-step guide on boosting self-esteem and how to apply it into your life moving forward. You will also learn other important things like listening to your inner voice and utilizing self-acceptance to live a happier life. Keep in mind that I can only provide you with the knowledge and tools, discipline and commitment is something you need to have in order to achieve your goal of living a more fulfilling life.

Chapter 1: Self-Esteem vs. Self-Confidence

You just learned the ins and outs of self-esteem and the importance it brings, now we will move onto learning more about self-confidence. Self-confidence often sounds very similar to self-esteem, but it is actually very different in its definition. The oxford dictionary definition of self-confidence is "a feeling of trust in one's abilities, qualities, and judgment". Unlike self-esteem, self-confidence is focused more on the way an individual performs and how that gives them the confidence to continue. When an individual is more confident in their ability to perform, they tend to be happier because of their successes. When an individual believes in their own capabilities, they become motivated to do the necessary things in order to achieve their goals. Self-confidence focuses on feeling good about past performances to create the power to improve future performance.

Just like self-esteem, self-confidence can be hard to understand properly. It is important to know what self-confidence actually means before we move on as it is a term that will be used consistently throughout this book and in your exercises. Below are a few examples that highlight the definition of self-confidence.

- An individual is able to value themselves for who they are disregarding past mistakes.
- An individual can feel good about themselves despite their imperfections and continue to value themselves as a person.
- An individual feeling brave enough to be assertive and to stand up for themselves.

- An individual knowing that they are worthy of respect and friendship from others.
- An individual is able to know and accept all aspects of themselves including both strengths and weaknesses.

Here is what self-confidence is NOT:
- An individual believing that they are perfect or having the belief that they should be perfect.
- An individual holding themselves to unrealistic expectations and standards.
- An individual striving for a life that does not have any problems, pains, or struggles.
- An individual being selfish and only care for their own goals and needs.

When first learning about self-confidence, many people confuse self-confidence with tunnel vision of only focusing on themselves so they can have an easier and smoother life. Although self-confidence does give you the tools you need to cope with problems that life throws at you, it absolutely does not mean that your life will be free of problems forever. Moreover, many people are under the impression that only focusing on your own goals and skill-building is an essential part of building self-confidence. However, what is being described is actually selfishness. People that are truly self-confident by definition are simply just confident in who they are as a person and what they can do for themselves and others. These behaviors described will make it more likely for the person to reach out and relate with others. Thus, this creates a more balanced and healthier life.

Now that we know what self-confidence is and isn't, how does it work in the real world? It's actually quite simple. Self-confidence works by helping you achieve healthy levels of self-esteem and helping you achieve confidence and love within yourself. When a person feels more confident in their ability to accomplish things, they will naturally be more successful. When they achieve success, they will gain the self-confidence needed to help motivate them to accomplish even more things and more goals. Even though there are many differences between self-esteem and self-confidence, they work as a team to help you create a healthy relationship with yourself.

Now, let's learn about some of the differences between self-confidence and self-esteem. As we have already learned, self-esteem is defined as the way a person feels about themselves and how much self-love they have. Self-esteem comes from the experiences and situations of one's life and they shape how that person views themselves in the present-day. Self-confidence is how a person feels and views their abilities and differs from situation to situation. For instance, I can have a healthy self-esteem but I have low self-confidence when it comes to my social skills. When a person shows themselves love, their self-esteem will increase which gives them more self-confidence to do new things. When an individual begins to feel confident in various areas of their life, they will slowly improve their overall self-esteem. These two concepts work together harmoniously so by improving your self-esteem, you can actually improve your self-confidence at the same time. Two birds, one stone.

So, what are the similarities between self-esteem and self-confidence? The main similarity here is that they both share the idea of the ability to love yourself. Many people that struggle with this likely have grown up in an environment where others did not value them which makes it very hard for these people to self-develop the ability to value themselves. When a person doesn't feel valued, their self-esteem will decrease. If they don't believe in themselves and their own abilities, they will then lack self-confidence. Just like how it is two birds with one stone, by not having self-esteem you will likely not have self-confidence in many areas of your life.

Just to summarize quickly, self-esteem is something that is developed through the events that the individual has experienced over their lifetime. Self-confidence is the ability where the individual values the things they do. Together, they form an important partnership within a person and is the biggest influencer on how a person feels about themselves, their overall level of confidence, and their assertiveness level. Here are a few tips that you can look over to begin improving your self-confidence and self-esteem.

- Try to remind yourself of the positive qualities that other people say you have. Even if you don't think they are right, just reminding yourself of them is the first step in the right direction.
- Try to mute the negative self-talk in your brain. Begin thinking of ways that you can contradict those comments.
- If you are having negative thoughts about yourself, ask yourself if those are things that you would say to a loved one? If not, stop yourself from thinking those thoughts.
- Make a list of your strengths. Imagine the things you would say about yourself during a job interview and add them to your list.

Chapter 2: Causes of Low Self-Esteem

People who suffer from low self-esteem often feel bad about who they are and constantly feel that they are inferior to others. Due to this, they are at risk of not fulfilling their true potential. They often don't take the initiative to set up and pursue their goals and may lead to not putting in effort into important things like their education and career. They may be prone to accepting bad treatment from people close to them like friends, significant others, and family. Research has associated these negative behaviors linked to low self-esteem in teens and adolescents:

- Teen pregnancy
- Criminal behavior
- Poor academic performance
- Dropping out of school
- Disordered eating
- Alcohol and drug abuse
- Earlier sexual activity

Having low self-esteem is more than just a negative feeling, it often takes a huge toll on people's lives. Although it's hard to determine how common low self-esteem is but many studies have found evidence that self-esteem levels drop dramatically for young people as they approach their teenagerhood. Many people in this demographic start to believe they aren't 'good enough' in aspects like school performance, relationships, and physical appearance.

When low self-esteem starts at a young age, it has a high chance of being carried into adulthood where it begins to interfere with one's ability to live a healthy and fulfilling life. An important thing to know about low self-esteem is that it is not an accurate reflection of reality, nor is it something that is set in stone. Sometimes the cause of low self-esteem can be found but the belief that your feelings regarding yourself cannot be changed is inaccurate.

Self-esteem is a mindset and can always be changed. Just like how someone who had healthy levels of self-esteem can change into having low levels of self-esteem, it can work the other way as well. A person can only improve their self-esteem if they are willing to acknowledge and challenge the negative judgments, they have about themselves. Regardless of how convinced they are of their current self-evaluation; they have nothing to lose but a world to gain by accepting the possibility that they have control over their own self-esteem. Making the conscious choice to challenge your own thinking can begin to change the way you think and what you do in the present and future.

Below we will learn about some of the common causes of low self-esteem in people and to help you discover the potential sources in your life that may be contributing to it.

Uninvolved or Negligent Parents

Almost everyone, especially when they are young, has feelings about themselves that heavily influenced by how the people closest to them treat them. This holds very true especially when it comes to their parents or guardians. Undoubtedly, everyone deserves to have a loving family but some people have the misfortune of not receiving the needed support. Often, it is the parents who suffer from mental health issues or other similar problems and challenges that are not able to give their children the guidance, attention and care that they need and deserve. This causes significant self-esteem problems for people at that age because the people responsible for them are not caring for them properly.

Negative Peers

Like the way low self-esteem individuals can be caused by the treatment from their parents/guardians, the way their peers treat them is also greatly influential. If an individual is a part of a social group that is constantly bringing them down, not respecting them, pressuring them to do things they are uncomfortable with and not valuing their thoughts and feelings can cause them to feel like something is wrong with them. It makes them feel like the only way for them to be liked is to do what others want and to disregard their own thoughts and opinions. This is very damaging to someone's self-esteem.

Trauma

Physical, emotion or sexual abuse often causes feelings of shame and guilt in a person. The individual may be under the impression that they did something to deserve this abuse or that they were not deserving of the love, care, and respect of the abuser. Individuals who have suffered through abuse may be affected by significant amounts of anxiety and depression that interfere with the ability to live a fulfilling life.

Body Image

Based on recent research, it was reported that about 50% of girls were not happy with the way their body looks and that number rises to almost 80% by the time they are 17 years old. In a similar study, it was reported that 30% of teenage boys and 50% of teenage girls would practice unhealthy behaviors to try to lose weight or to achieve the body they want. These unhealthy behaviors included skipping meals, smoking cigarettes, using laxatives, fasting, and vomiting.

In a young person's self-esteem, body image plays a huge role, especially in women. From the moment that we were born, we have been surrounded by unrealistic images of what women should look like and what body type is most 'ideal'. Women's bodies are one of the most objectified things in media and it gives the impression that women's bodies exist for the purpose of others to touch, look at, and use. When puberty takes place and girl's bodies begin to change, they don't see the things they see in the media and often leads to them feeling unattractive on top of the feeling of powerlessness that is associated with viewing your body as an object for others to use.

Young men are also not immune to having a bad body image. Many of them struggle with the same things women do, like weight and body composition. However, young men are more affected by their concern about muscle mass. Different from women, however, the man's body is not treated as an object for other people but rather as a symbol of masculinity. Young boys often feel pressured to develop big muscles to show off their strength and masculinity and they often feel insecure about their height.

Small Fish, Big Pond

It is not hard for people at a young age to feel like they are uncontrollably being swallowed up by the whole world. This creates feelings of powerlessness, worthlessness, and ineffectiveness. Most young people don't experience these feelings until adulthood, but it is very possible for younger people to go through the famous "existential crisis". This is a time where the meaning of one's life is questioned. Questions like 'what really matters?' and "what is my purpose?" are asked and the inability to find answers poses a big threat to a person's sense of self-worth.

Unrealistic Goals

When individuals face pressure from themselves or other people like their peers or authority figures, some individuals may expect too much of themselves in terms of achievement in school, extracurriculars, and social status. Those who are struggling with their academics may believe that they need to get straight A's all the time while those who perform well in their academics may try to take on too many other activities and expect that they will also be the best at them. Those people who seek popularity may be worried that not everyone likes them and wants everyone to like them even though that is impossible as no matter who you are, it isn't possible to please everybody. The inevitability of failure to meet those unrealistic goals leads to the feeling of overall failure.

Previous Bad Choices

Many people get stuck in a specific pattern of acting and decision making. It could be because this individual wasn't a very good friend in the past or they didn't pay attention in school or they participated in dangerous behaviors like unprotected sex or drug use. They may believe to think that they are just 'that kind of person' who acts in those unhealthy ways. They may even start to dislike themselves because of bad decisions in the past and don't seem to believe that they can change their path now so, therefore, they don't try. They may continue to make choices that purposely reinforces the negative way that they view themselves.

Negative Thought Patterns

When people get used to the way they think, feel, and talk about themselves, it automatically becomes a habit. Just like muscle memory, when you perform a specific physical act like swimming repeatedly, your brain automatically signals your muscles to do the things that the activity requires. People's feelings and thoughts work the exact same way. If you feel worthless or inferior frequently, you will constantly continue to think negative thoughts about yourself and you are more likely to live your life feeling and thinking that way until you can break the cycle by challenging those thoughts. Just like our muscle memory can learn an incorrect way of performing a physical act, our feelings can learn incorrect patterns as well.

These causes of self-esteem are not the only ones out there but just the most common ones that are studied. Cause #8 (Negative Thought Patterns) is responsible for the persistence of low self-esteem in most people and doesn't consider what the initial causes were. The people who suspect that they are suffering from low self-esteem should look into situations in their lives at home, school, and social circles to help identify potential sources of low self-esteem.

Chapter 3: Benefits of Boosting Self-Esteem

Now that we have learned about some of the negative effects of low self-esteem and its causes, we will be learning about the benefits that come with increasing your self-esteem. As we have learned, self-esteem and self-confidence directly affect one another and without a good level of self-esteem, it is almost impossible to create the necessary self-confidence that is required to achieve the things that you want to do in life. By learning the benefits of having healthy self-esteem, you can begin to feel motivated enough to start practicing techniques to help you improve your self-esteem. Bear in mind that although it is more difficult to increase self-esteem later in life, it is not entirely impossible. It requires hard work like practicing self-awareness, mindfulness, and self-awareness. If you are someone who is planning to have children or already have children, keep in mind that self-esteem is extremely impressionable in the growing up stages of a child's life. Be mindful of how you are treating your children and remember how important it is to make a child growing up feel important and valued. Having this base of self-esteem will give them a healthy level of self-esteem later in life so that they can be confident in who they are and their ability to achieve goals in the future. Let's dive into the benefits of having a healthy self-esteem.

Self-Esteem Increases Your Assertiveness When Expressing Your Thoughts and Needs

Assertiveness is something that is absolutely required to live a healthy life. Having self-esteem helps with this by creating a strong belief in the things you are saying, doing, and asking. If an individual believes that they need or want something, they often don't spend any time dwelling on if people think it is true, instead, they just ask for it. Individuals that have low self-esteem often have trouble with assertiveness because of the fear of being rejected or judged. They often think that asking for something they need is a sign of weakness and therefore, they will be judged for simply asking. On the other hand, an individual with healthy self-esteem isn't afraid of asking for what they need because that thought of doubt simply doesn't cross their mind. Having healthy self-esteem comes from the root of loving and respecting yourself and those who have it, it feels very normal to ask for what they want and need.

To explain more in-depth about the meaning of assertiveness, I will provide you with an example. Imagine if your mother asked you to go over to her house as soon as you can to help her move and pack her things. However, you had already planned to spend your evening doing relaxing things like taking a hot bath and watching a light-hearted movie since you had a rough week at work. What assertiveness means, in this case, is being able to value your own needs as much as you value your mother's. A person that has healthy self-esteem will be assertive by saying to themselves "I am worthy and deserving of this break because I need it." A person with low self-esteem may say "It is selfish of me to take a break when somebody I love is asking for my help." A fundamental part of having healthy self-esteem is understanding that you cannot pour from a glass that is empty. In this example, if the person has low self-esteem they will likely go and help their mother move despite being very fatigued and will end up feeling like their time and feelings are not respected by others. However, people do not know how other people feel until they communicate it so the mother is not at fault for simply asking.

Here's one more example of assertiveness, this time the example will be in the place of work. Imagine if your manager just asked you for the fourth time this month to step in and complete your co-worker's deliverable because she has fallen behind schedule yet once again and knows that you are a more efficient employee than her. Someone with healthy self-esteem will respond with assertiveness like "This is the fourth time in the month that I have taken on extra work because Jessica is behind schedule, again. I highly value being a team player but I feel stressed when I am overwhelmed with extra work. What can we do to make sure this doesn't happen so often?" That is the ideal way to respond to your manager in a situation like this because you have to have enough respect yourself to tell them that enough is enough. A person with low self-esteem in this situation will likely agree to take on the extra work and end up resenting their coworker for it. They may drain themselves too much by doing more work and blame other people for it thus creating unhealthy relationships. By communicating with others to let them know your feelings and needs will give them an opportunity to understand and adjust their own actions accordingly.

Learning to be assertive is a life skill that is important due to how often it is used and respected. If you think you are suffering from the "yes" syndrome, your first step may be to work on your self-esteem to help you respect your own wants and needs. In this book, you will be provided with multiple worksheets and exercises that aid you in expressing your needs and learning to be assertive. Take into consideration however, that being assertive is not the same as being aggressive. Many people avoid being assertive as they confuse it with aggression. Assertiveness means to be firm and clear about what one needs/wants while aggression is a harsh demand. The way you deliver your message using body language and tone of voice influences how people perceive your request.

Self-Esteem Increases Your Confidence in Decision-Making

The second benefit of having self-esteem is the ability to improve the confidence that is required when it comes to decision-making. Since a person's life is mainly determined by the decisions they make, those who have low self-esteem are affected by the anxiety of that truth. Having self-esteem allows a person to recognize their needs, wants and their own respect for them. This makes the process of decision making easier since you understand your goal and are dedicated to making a decision that makes it easier for you to achieve that goal. People with low self-esteem often spend hours contemplating and playing out every scenario of failure. They become caught up in the nervousness about what others might say or think about their decision.

To give you a deeper understanding, here are a few consequences that come with the lack of confidence in decision making:

- **Decision-Making Paralysis**
  People who have low self-esteem often avoid making decisions because they become so overwhelmed in the process. This will get people stuck in the same place in life as they prefer to stay where they are than risk making the wrong decision. Those who are guilty of this may feel lousy about themselves.

- **Zero Trust in Made Decisions**
  Those who have low self-esteem have trouble believing that the decision they made was the best for the specific situation. They will begin to convince themselves that another decision should have been made.

- **Refusal to Take Charge**
  In certain situations where large decisions need to be made, a person with low self-esteem may prefer to offload that responsibility to someone else. This way, they can rest easy because they believe someone else would be able to make a better decision. They think that because they are less intelligent and capable that it makes sense for someone better to help them with that decision. Then, in the scenario that things go south due to that decision, they can easily blame the other person.

- **Shrinking Life Options**
  Those with low self-esteem may find themselves with limited options in life that are continually shrinking. They are more likely to miss out on opportunities that would potentially work out for them. For example, one could think their current position at their current job is as far as they can go in their career while others may find you capable of achieving greater things. Since they imposed limits on themselves, they find it hard to have the motivation to pursue promotions or new challenges.

By teaching you the consequences of having low confidence regarding decision making, I hope that it will motivate you to improve your self-esteem in order to improve your confidence when it comes to decision making. Having the required self-esteem to make decisions confidently will provide an individual with the maximum amount of opportunity and build trust in oneself when making decisions regarding themselves. The fundamentals of making decisions grow from self-esteem so by starting to love and respect yourself you are taking the right step forward. You may find that once you have a clear idea of what your needs, wants, and goals are, your decision making will become easier. For example, say an individual is working on their self-esteem and has been doing many worksheets and they discover that what they want is a successful career, enough rest and to achieve a promotion by the end of the year. If they are faced with the decision of whether or not they should go on an extended vacation in November, they can properly assess their goals to make a decision that makes the most sense. Based on their wants, needs, and goals, the decision that benefits them most is to book this vacation in the new year instead so they can keep working towards their main goal of achieving a promotion at the end of the year. They can then also celebrate with a well-deserved vacation despite the result of their promotion.

Self-Esteem Helps You Feel Secure, Safe, And Honest in Relationships

There is a famous saying that says 'you must learn to love yourself before you can love other people'. This holds a lot of truth on the topic we are about to discuss. One of the main benefits of having self-esteem is the ability to show love and respect for yourself. This means that you won't be likely to seek out love and respect from others unhealthily. You will feel more secure and safe in relationships due to valuing yourself as a person.

In recent research, scientists have found evidence that confirms the relationship between healthy self-esteem and relationship satisfaction. We already learned about how self-esteem affects the way an individual thinks and feels about themselves but it also affects the amount of love they are capable of receiving. It also has a big effect on how individuals treat other people in intimate relationships. A person's level of self-esteem before entering a relationship can predict the overall relationship satisfaction between the two people. Although happiness in relationships generally declines slowly over time (naturally) this is false for those who enter a relationship with a good amount of self-esteem. It's been proven that when people with low self-esteem enter a relationship, they have the steepest decline in happiness overall. These relationships also have the tendency to not last. Even though communication, stress, and emotionality are all factors that contribute to the final outcome of a relationship, an individual's self-esteem and experiences all play a role in how they manage those issues. Therefore, self-esteem affects the outcome of a relationship the most amongst all other factors.

Now your next question may be how does a person's self-esteem affect their relationships? Earlier in the book, we discussed how self-esteem suffers dramatically if a person had a dysfunctional childhood. Individuals who have gone through these experiences feel like not only are they not valued but they don't have a voice when it comes to anything. Their opinions, wants, and needs are often not acknowledged and if they are, they aren't taken seriously. In cases like this, the parents may also have low self-esteem and are in an unhappy relationship. These parents often may not have had a good role model, relationship skills, healthy boundaries, assertiveness, and cooperation. Some may even be nearing on the abusive end and exhibiting controlling, manipulative, and preoccupied behavior. This may cause them to shame the way their children feel and judge them for their personality traits.

This will result in the child feeling like they are emotionally abandoned and are forced to draw conclusions that he/she is not good enough to be accepted and respected by their parents and that it is their fault. Children who grow up feeling anxious, insecure, and unsafe to be themselves often end up in codependent relationships.

Individuals who grew up in dysfunctional families typically exhibit low self-esteem which is unhealthy within relationships. They tend to develop an anxious or avoidant attachment style that is caused by feelings of shame, insecurity, and low self-esteem. People who have avoidant and anxious attachments often showcase behaviors of pursuers and distancers. In some scenarios, people who have these behaviors struggle to be too close or too alone. Either one creates pain for them. The anxiety that they feel can lead them to give up their own needs to please someone else's. Resulting from basic insecurity, this person may be completely occupied by their relationship and is tuned completely to their partner and they may begin to worry that the other person wants space. Since their needs aren't being met as they haven't done anything to care for themselves, they become unhappy. It then begins to snowball where they begin to take things too personally and actively projecting negative outcomes. Having low self-esteem tends to make a person hide their feelings and thoughts in order to not 'dump on the other person' which compromises intimacy. They will begin to feel jealousy when their partner is giving attention to others and after attempts of seeking reassurance, they will unintentionally push their significant other away. This is the process behind how low self-esteem is related to unsuccessful relationships.

However, those who have healthy self-esteem allow the opportunity for deep intimacy with their significant other which gives them the opportunity to take care of you as well. Those with healthy self-esteem don't face problems like avoidance, abandonment issues, and anxiety. Since their needs are met and they feel fulfilled, they are comfortable spending more or less time with their partner. They understand that fulfilling their own needs first comes before attending to others. They are comfortable expressing genuine feelings to their partner and feel comfortable hearing theirs as well. Jealousy tends to not be an issue at all as you trust yourself and your partner since they have not done anything to prove otherwise. This is the reason why people with healthy self-esteem enter relationships constantly find success. They are proving the saying of 'learning to love yourself before you can love anybody else' true.

Self-Esteem Lowers the Likelihood of Staying in An Unhealthy Relationship

As we just learned, self-esteem helps people feel safe, secure, and honest when in relationships. It also helps you realize when the relationship you are in is unhealthy. The concept here is very straightforward; if an individual has a healthy amount of self-esteem, they are able to identify their wants, needs, and opinions and will prioritize those when making decisions. However, if an individual has low self-esteem, they are unable to identify their own wants and needs but will be unable to prioritize them. The dictionary definition of an unhealthy relationship is where at least one person in the relationship shows unhealthy behaviors and does not come from a place of respect for the other person.

Those that have a healthy level of self-esteem are able to realize and ask for things when they realize that their own needs are not being met. If the individual is able to realize this, they are able to let their partner know with an assertiveness that something needs to change or the relationship will not last. On the contrary, someone with low self-esteem does not have the ability to ask for what they need because they are unable to recognize what their needs are. They also lack the skills needed to be assertive with their partner to let them know that they need a change in the relationship. People with low self-esteem often have the mindset of them not doing enough or doing things right and that is the reason why their significant other isn't happy. They don't stop often enough to think for themselves.

If you are someone that is in a relationship right now and you feel like you are dealing with symptoms of low self-esteem, don't worry. This book is here to help you discover some of the meanings and reasons behind the way things are in your life. You will be provided with various tips, tricks, and exercises to help you fight the symptoms of low self-esteem. Below is a checklist of relationship behaviors that are normally exhibited in people with low self-esteem. Check off the ones that apply to you. This exercise is meant to help you see which areas in your relationships you need to focus more on.

Negative Relationship Behavior Checklist

- **Being Clingy/Needy**
  When someone has insecurities that run very deep, they often feel that they don't deserve love or that their significant other may break up with them at any moment, they may be exhibiting symptoms of needy behavior. The harder somebody tries to hold on to something, the more likely it is for them to drive it further away instead.

- **Apologizing for Your Existence**
  The purpose of an apology is to let the person you've wronged know that you are sorry. If an individual finds themselves apologizing over almost everything that they do, it could be reflecting your sense of self-worth.

- **Asking for Permission**
  If a person is asking for permission around every little thing they do such as visiting family, buying food to eat, or simply just pausing the TV, they are likely seeking approval or is a victim to a controlling relationship. The person may be looking for validation due to their low self-esteem.

- **Being A People Pleaser**
  One of the major symptoms of low self-esteem is being a people pleaser. These individuals try their best to be extra kind and overly helpful because they feel the necessity to prove their worth. They often don't feel comfortable with conflict so they always try their best to keep their partner happy while disregarding their own feelings.

- **Co-dependence**
  Co-dependence occurs when people in a relationship both have low self-esteem. Codependency is when the two people rely on each other far too much. It can range from setting up your life around the other person or feeling the inability to live without them. People with healthy self-esteem are able to maintain their individuality.

- **Distance**
  When individuals in a relationship feel a distance from their partner it is likely stemmed from low self-esteem

and trust issues. People use distance as a type of self-defense in order to shield themselves from getting hurt by not letting people get close to them in the first place.

- **Enabling**
  Individuals that have low self-esteem may start doing unhealthy things all for the sake of satisfying their significant other. This could be in the form of enablement. Enablement includes helping the other person solve all their problems or gifting them money for their addictions.

- **Oversensitivity**
  If an individual is often crying or upset at their significant other for the things they said (even if it was lighthearted) it is likely a symptom of low self-esteem. Lighthearted questions like "did you order food delivery tonight for dinner or did you cook this?" may cause the other person to be thrown into a spiral of "they hate my cooking!" or "my cooking sucks!" although their partner said nothing amongst those lines.

- **Lying**
  When an individual has low self-esteem, they may make lies about themselves to be more like the person they want to be, not who they actually are. They may go as far as trying to become the person that their partner wants them to be.

- **Not Setting Boundaries**
  People who have low self-esteem often are terrified of their partner leaving them which causes them the inability to communicate when their partner treats them in a way that they don't like. They tend to accept

all and any type of behavior from them even if they know it isn't good.

- **Not Making Decisions**
  If an individual avoids making decisions because they are afraid that their partner won't like it, this is a sign of low self-esteem. They need to keep in mind that their opinions are real and valid just like theirs.

Self-Esteem Helps You Develop Realistic Expectations of Yourself and Others

Throughout a person's life, we all have set unrealistic expectations for ourselves. For example, some people strive to be in the Olympics at the age of 18 without any prior athletic experience or they might want to be a millionaire by the ripe age of 22. The main difference between these unrealistic expectations set by people with low self-esteem versus people with high self-esteem is that those with low self-esteem will judge themselves harshly when an unrealistic expectation is not achieved. A part of having healthy self-esteem is it helps a person develop realistic expectations for themselves because they are aware of what their abilities are. By being able to understand your own abilities, they can set goals based on their skills, lifestyle, and resources. Therefore, they can make a plan that reflects their goals and needs. However, if an individual has low self-esteem, they often spend more time and energy focusing on what other people have achieved and they often feel like they will never be able to measure up. Rather than spending time developing their own plan and goals, they often spend that time self-loathing and wondering why they haven't reached the same goals as the people they are comparing themselves to. They begin to dwell in self-pity and blame external factors. For instance, they may blame their financial situation, their family, or their surrounding environment. Those factors obviously still have a huge role in a person's ability to achieve their goals but those with healthy self-esteem spend their focus on problem-solving rather than stopping altogether due to one obstacle.

To explain this further, here are a few common examples of unrealistic expectations that people have. Remember these as you begin to make your own goals throughout this workbook.

- "Life should be fair and equal for everyone!" The common saying that 'life isn't fair' holds very true in this expectation. Although yes, life SHOULD be fair, it, unfortunately, isn't. It is necessary to move past that harsh reality.
- "Opportunities will present themselves to me!" People must realize that the opportunity doesn't just present itself to anyone. Just because you believe you deserve a certain opportunity does not mean it will be handed to you. You must go out in the world and work towards getting what you want.
- "Everyone should be like me!" Even though an individual may be wonderful and amazing, not everyone else in the world is going to be the same way. Don't have the expectations that other people will treat you in the way that you will treat them.
- "Everyone should agree with me!" Although there are numerous answers to one question, nothing in this world is black and white so expect people to have different opinions in the grey area.
- "I'm always going to fail!" There are so many studies that have proven that having a successful mindset leads to a higher chance of succeeding. This holds true for having a mindset of failure. Change your mindset to a more positive one if you are serious about your goals.

Here are a few realistic expectations that you can learn instead:

- Expect to need help from others at some point. Achieving goals without the help of others is often unrealistic especially if your goals are big. Instead, replace it with the mindset that you will likely require help along the way. This will motivate you to build stronger relationships with people.
- Expect failure along the way. It is impossible for a person to achieve their goals in a smooth fashion. Everyone experiences failure along the way. Accept that fact now so you aren't surprised with that truth later.
- Expect to have to improve your own skills and abilities. Don't be under the impression that your goals are achievable just by remaining the same way you are now. If it is a big goal, it will likely require you to learn new skills or develop existing ones.
- Expect the goal to change your reality when you reach it. Just because someone reached their biggest goal does not mean their life will be perfect afterward. Their reality will change which means they will be faced with new problems and obstacles, this is normal.

Think of these realistic expectations the next time you are setting your goals. By being more forgiving of your failures and learning to accept help from others will help you reach your goals more successfully. Try offering help to other people with their goals to help yourself realize that asking for help or giving help from others is the opposite of failing.

Self-Esteem Increases Resilience to Stress and Obstacles

Scientific studies have shown a relationship between having healthy self-esteem to less stress overall. Since self-esteem impacts your happiness level directly, it also largely contributes to how a person feels about their life. If one is able to trust their ability to move past obstacles, they will view difficult situations as a challenge and not as a threat. However, if a person isn't able to trust their own ability to deal with stressful circumstances, they will likely see them as stress-inducing and threatening. Self-efficacy is the dictionary term that describes a person's ability to feel resourceful and capable. Self-efficacy is another component that plays a role in stress management and self-esteem.

Since the relationship between self-esteem and stress has been proven, they tend to feed off each other and act out in many ways. When a person has low self-esteem, it causes them to have negative psychological experiences that make them more prone to stress. A person with healthy self-esteem that is always dealing with consistent stress in their life can have their self-esteem lowered over time. However, having healthy self-esteem allows a person to use it as protection against stress while environments with low stress levels are more comfortable for people who lack self-esteem.

The dictionary definition of stress is "feeling of pressure and/or worry". One thing that people need to understand is that the main determining factor of the level of stress that a person is feeling is based on how they perceive the situation and now just the actual circumstances of the situation. Let's use moving homes as an example here. Person A may see moving their homes as an exciting opportunity to start somewhere new while person B may see it as a huge trouble.

The difference of perception between person A and person B is dependent on their level of self-esteem and how they view their own abilities to move homes.

The connection between self-esteem and stress is more damaging to people that have low self-esteem. They often feel negative emotions like powerlessness, incapability, and helplessness. They often feel incapable of overcoming obstacles and tend to think that any task, no matter how simple or difficult, is impossible and even daily routine tasks seem challenging.

Chapter 4: Benefits of Boosting Self-Confidence

Just like self-esteem, there are also many benefits to be gained by boosting self-confidence. At this point, we've learned that if self-esteem is increased it naturally increases the level of self-confidence as well. Since self-confidence has a more external effect in comparison to self-esteem, its benefits tend to be more external as well. Often times, people are capable of hiding their low self-esteem, but self-confidence is more difficult to hide. Discovering that a person has low self-esteem comes from getting to know them through conversations and being around them for a long time. On the other hand, discovering that a person has low self-confidence can be easy just by analyzing their social ability, comfort, and physical posture. By boosting self-confidence, a person will be able to change the outcomes of their actions and gain respect and admiration for other people. Self-confidence is very important for people who work in a team environment. When a person has more self-confidence, they will be able to foster a more collaborative working environment where they are able to express their opinions and ideas rather than taking a backseat and going along with other people's suggestions. The ability to diplomatically share their thoughts and opinions is a highly sought after leadership quality that many successful people have. Here are the benefits of having higher self-confidence:

Increasing Self-Confidence Increases Overall Performance

When self-confidence is increased, it is directly related to better overall performance. For example, when a person first starts to play a new sport or video game, they naturally get better the more they practice. When a person starts something brand new, on the first day they may have lower self-confidence. However, when they start getting better at it, they naturally develop more confidence when they realize that their skills have improved. This example is exactly how self-confidence affects a person's overall performance in everything. People who start new things with higher confidence levels tend to be better at it right at the beginning compared to those who have lower self-confidence.

People like actors, athletes, public speakers, and entrepreneurs understand the importance of self-confidence. They know that if they lack confidence, it can get in their way of achieving their peak performance. They also know that if they have confidence, they can easily solve problems to work past obstacles to continue striving for their goal. One effective trick that personal trainers or coaches use in the gym when they are training their clients with weightlifting is to manipulate their mindset to help them feel more confident. For instance, if a weightlifter's personal record with deadlifts is 80kg, the personal trainer will tell them that the weight they are lifting now is 80kg when in fact the trainer had secretly added an extra 10kg weight on their barbell making it 90kg. With the client under the mindset that they have already lifted 80kg before, they believe that they can do it and most likely they will be able to pull off lifting 90kg. If they do it and they succeed, the personal trainer will tell them that they had actually lifted 10kg above their personal record. However, if the personal trainer had told them before the exercise that they will be lifting 90kg instead of 80kg, the client may be intimidated or feel unconfident at that number and therefore fail to achieve that lift due to their mindset. This trick is used frequently in the world of athletics and gives us proof that a positive and confident mindset is more important than your hard skills.

Increasing Self-Confidence Increases Overall Happiness

When a person has a healthy amount of self-confidence, they will naturally feel more confident when completing tasks which leads them to have a higher success rate. Therefore, they feel good and confident in themselves which leads to higher happiness. People who work in Confidence Building programs and workshops often report that the people who are happier and have more life satisfaction usually exhibit more self-confidence.

People that have more self-confidence tend to take on the world with intensity and conviction which helps them feel more connected with their environment and feel more satisfied in relationships. Naturally, they also have higher influential ability and have the skills to manage their emotions and behaviors in a more compelling way. Due to this, successful leaders usually have higher self-confidence which automatically gains respect from their followers which fosters a healthy and functional team environment. Self-confidence is exactly like self-esteem in the sense that feeling good about yourself and your abilities create a positive attitude.

One of the most misunderstood things in the world is where happiness comes from. Often, when humans are asked what they think will make them happier, their answers tend to be:

- A significant other
- More money
- A child

- More time
- Buying a better house
- Buying a better car
- Getting a better job

The common element between all those answers is that they are simply things. Owning things or having things does not lead to happiness. Often it is actually the opposite where having too many things actually leads to less happiness. What drives a person's happiness is the ability to understand their inner self and living in harmony with it. By understanding the things that are actually important to you, you will know how to go and achieve it. Self-confidence is the driving factor that helps you achieve these things. By aiming to have the things in the list above, you need to have self-confidence in knowing the changes and sacrifices you need to make in order to attain them. If you don't have confidence regarding this, you will likely feel helpless and wonder why life isn't fair and that you are unable to have the things that other people have.

Increasing Self-Confidence Increases Social Ability

In social situations, people that have healthy self-confidence levels tend to be more relaxed especially during the interaction when meeting someone new. When self-confidence is at a healthy level, an individual's belief in themselves is internal and is not affected by other people's judgments. People like this can move freely within social situations without fearing rejection. Psychologists say that self-confidence helps create a sensation of comfort when someone is faced with a new challenge. People who are self-confident feel excited about their future and are comfortable expressing that excitement with other people. Since they feel confident and excited, they can carry themselves that way and converse with more ease and excitement. Due to this, confident people feel more at ease in most social situations and this attribute draws attention from others. The positive energy that this person exhibits is very contagious and desirable to other people.

Others have the argument that having confidence in social settings is more valued than having confidence in hard skills. Important parts of our lives like jobs and opportunities are often rewarded to those with exceptional social skills. Lots of recent research discuss that modern employers value a person's emotional intelligence over their IQ. When hiring managers are comparing a candidate with more experience but less emotional intelligence to a candidate with less experience but more emotional intelligence, the most popular choice is the person that has more social skills and ease. This is valued more due to how important the human connection is in most workplaces. A person's confidence directly affects their ability to build and develop relationships. Therefore, since most jobs require human interaction, the person who can develop and build the most effective relationships is more likely to succeed.

Due to our natural human instinct, most people feel more attracted to people that exhibit more self-confidence. Back in the day, our ancestors that had the best physique are likely the ones that had more self-confidence. Those who had both attributes, physical fitness, and good self-confidence usually had the role of a leader and therefore, more people were attracted to them. As we evolved to our present day, our attraction to physical looks may have changed but our attraction towards confidence didn't. People continue to be drawn to those who have confident behavior and they respect them more naturally. Don't worry, if you feel like you are someone who lacks self-confidence, this book will provide you with enough worksheets and exercises that you can do to help boost your self-confidence to exhibit those attractive behaviors.

Improving Self-Confidence Improves Physical and Mental Health

Healthy self-esteem and self-confidence are the main indicators of good mental wellbeing according to the National Mental Health Centre. As we already learned, healthy self-esteem in the early stages comes from a person's childhood where their parents help build their character and confidence level. Children that grew up in a positive and encouraging environment have more confidence and tend to do better in school, excelling in sports, social skills, and generally take care of themselves better. When children grow into their teenagerhood, those with healthy self-confidence handle peer pressure better and can make good decisions based on their best interests.

Under the theory of the mind and body connection, it proposes that a person's physical health affects their mental health and vice versa. People who suffer from disorders like anxiety and depression tend to have lowered physical health such as a weaker immune system or chronic pains. Taking care of yourself physically like eating healthy and exercising can help improve health but having good mental health can prevent physical problems in general.

Individuals who have good physical health typically also have higher happiness as they can do more things within their life. They have more energy and motivation to get out in the world and accomplish things or simply just to socialize. Humans naturally feed off other human's happiness so if a person is spending time with someone who is confident and happy, it is can be beneficial for them. This is why you often see people that are confident in the same social circles. People with good mental health are attracted to those who have the same and prefer to dedicate their time to those people rather than others who don't showcase the same traits.

Chapter 5: Recognizing Your Level of Self-Esteem

At this point in the book, you have learned the fundamentals of self-esteem, self-confidence and all the benefits that come with it. Just to refresh your memory, self-esteem is the opinion that you have of yourself. When a person has healthy self-esteem, they feel good about who they are and feel worthy of respect. When a person has low self-esteem, they don't value their own thoughts and opinions as much. In order to help you build your self-esteem, we first must identify how much self-esteem you have. In this chapter, you will learn what the different ranges of self-esteem are and what comes with each level.

A person's self-esteem fluctuates throughout their life depending on their circumstances or stage of life. It is nor out of the ordinary to have moments where a person feels down about themselves and not strange to have moments where they feel good about themselves. Generally, a person's self-esteem stays within a range that relates directly to their opinion of themselves and is known to increase as a person gets older. The range here is low self-esteem to high self-esteem. Healthy self-esteem is located right in between the two extremes. The ideal level here is to have self-esteem somewhere in the middle and not aim to have 'high' self-esteem. This is called boasting and often is just a cover-up for having low self-esteem. However, for our purposes let's consider high self-esteem as its own extreme and not just another type of low self-esteem.

How to Recognize If You Have Low Self-Esteem

The people who don't value their own thoughts and opinions tend to have low self-esteem. They often don't focus on their own skills and credit that they deserve but instead focuses on their past mistakes and perceived weaknesses. They tend to have the mindset that other people are better or more capable than them. They also struggle with accepting positive feedback. They find themselves being afraid of failure which prevents them from trying to do things and ultimately, holds them back from success.

Below is a checklist of symptoms showcased in a person who has low self-esteem. Please check off the ones you think you exhibit. If four or more boxes are checked off, you are likely to have low self-esteem.

- ❑ You are doubtful in your ability to reach success.
- ❑ You choose the wrong partners for you.
- ❑ You criticize other people often.
- ❑ You are afraid of being alone.
- ❑ You become rigid.
- ❑ You always put the needs of other people before your own.
- ❑ You often feel ashamed.
- ❑ You experience regular anxiety.
- ❑ You often feel depressed.

If you notice that you exhibit a lot of these behaviors in the list above, that is totally fine. We will soon be diving into the worksheets and exercises that will help you boost your self-esteem.

How to Recognize If You Have Healthy Self-Esteem

People who have an overall positive opinion of themselves tend to have healthy self-esteem. Rather than dwelling on past or future failures, they believe in their ability to achieve goals. They are not scared of asking for help and they exert assertiveness in situations where it does not suit their best interests.

By focusing on past achievements and goals of future achievement, people with healthy self-esteem have more overall happiness in life because they are not dwelling on past mistakes or failures. Having confidence helps an individual be better at most life-related tasks and in sports or social situations. These people make a commitment to themselves to always put themselves first before trying to please anyone else.

Here is a checklist of behaviors that are exhibited by a person with healthy self-esteem. Check off the ones you think you exhibit. If you have <4 boxes checked off you are likely to have low to medium self-esteem if you have >4 boxes checked off, you are likely to have medium-high self-esteem.

- You live your life with humility.
- You can differentiate between the past and present.
- You take accountability when you commit to doing something.
- You speak the truth as you see it, without being afraid of rejection and without malicious intent.
- You can deliver a message to someone with your personal feelings put aside.
- You can identify where anger, guilt, fear, or any other negative emotions come from.

- You don't follow others just because other people are doing it.
- You believe in your own and other people's decision-making ability.

What did you find your results to be? Do you have healthier self-esteem or less self-esteem than you thought? This book will have enough exercises in the later chapters to suit the needs of all self-esteem levels.

How to Recognize If You Have High Self Esteem

As we discussed earlier in this chapter, it is arguable that people with high self-esteem actually is trying to cover up for the fact that they have low self-esteem. High self-esteem is very different than healthy self-esteem because a person with a healthy self-esteem does not exhibit traits of conceitedness or cockiness. People with healthy self-esteem actually exhibit traits opposite to that like humility and modesty. Rather than earning respect from others, those with high self-esteem don't respect themselves enough so they need to make up for it by over-communicating their strengths and skills with the intention of getting others to show them the respect they want. In other words, this is overcompensation.

Even though people with high self-esteem actually have low self-esteem, they tend to have behaviors that differ from those with low self-esteem. To put things simply, an individual with low self-esteem does not believe in their own capabilities when it comes to accomplishing tasks and therefore shies away from most things or relies on others to do it for them. Individuals with high self-esteem similarly also don't believe in their capabilities of accomplishing tasks and also shies away from it, but they don't hide their inabilities by avoiding the task, instead, they hide it by the usage of words to brag about their skills and abilities. There is a clear difference here.

Individuals that have healthy self-esteem do not usually exhibit the behaviors of bragging or boasting. Instead, these people have confidence when they are speaking about a topic that they have accomplishments. Those with high self-esteem often bring up parts of their life with the intention of bragging about it in order to mask their low self-esteem in other parts of their life. For instance, person A that has healthy self-esteem may say "After 2 years of training for the triathlon and failing the past couple times, I finally was able to finish it! I am now training for the next 20 weeks for the Iron Man competition." Person A is expressing how proud they feel regarding the work that they have put into their success without leaving out the obstacles they faced during their journey. On the contrary, person B with low self-esteem may sound like this "I only trained for 6 months and finished the triathlon while other people take years to train for it! I bet I could've done it without any training at all." The difference in the statement that person B made is that they are not talking about the obstacles and failures that they have faced along the way. We know that avoiding failure is impossible, so their statement is likely not truthful. They also focused on comparing themselves with other people where a person with a healthy self-esteem doesn't compare their own achievements with others.

Below is another checklist of behaviors. This time it is showcasing the behaviors of a person with high self-esteem. Check off the ones that apply to you.

- You often don't take on projects or opportunities because you think that they are too "easy" or you deem them as beneath your abilities.

- You take on too many projects when you full on know that you don't have the skills to finish all of them.
- You often notice some distance between you and some of your friends and suspect that it may be related to your possible arrogance.
- You notice some people seem put off at work and you suspect it may be due to you acting overly conceited.
- You find that you are more concerned with your own skills and performance and are not involved with your partners at all.

If you have checked off a few of those behaviors, that is totally fine! Your high self-esteem is probably a mask for low self-esteem. There will be plenty of practices throughout this book to boost your self-esteem to a healthy level.

Chapter 6: 10 Steps and Exercises to Boost Self-Esteem

In this chapter, we are going to be diving into the actual exercises and worksheets to help people boost their self-esteem or even to just maintain their healthy level of self-esteem. Keep in mind that you shouldn't be judging yourself if you have low self-esteem but accept it as what it is. Most people's self-esteem was developed by factors that they could not control in their childhood. By taking charge and diving into worksheets and exercises, you are well on your way to rebuilding it.

Step 1: Visualization

The first step in increasing one's self-esteem is to practice visualization. This exercise helps the person see a better image of themselves that they can be proud of within their own minds. Those who have low self-esteem often are trapped with having a negative image of themselves in their mind that is far from accurate. Visualization is an excellent technique to get used to seeing yourself achieving goals.

Worksheet #6.1

Visualizing a Positive You

In this exercise, write down in the lines below a few of your positive qualities and a description of a positive version of you looks like.

Ex: I am humble, hardworking, and generous. A positive me looks like someone who is trying their best to help other people that need it. I work hard every day to achieve my goals and I don't boast about my accomplishments. I don't try to avoid challenges and I am comfortable with asking for help when I am faced with them.

____

____

____

____

____

____

____

____

Was it easy or difficult for you to visualize a positive you? People often struggle thinking of positive things about themselves during this exercise and find it difficult to envision themselves in a positive way. This is because when a person has low self-esteem, they tend to only be aware of their negative experiences which confirms their own negative outlook on themselves. People may not pay attention to the good things that they have achieved, their desirable qualities, or the positive compliments given by other people. This makes it hard for an individual to be able to come up with positive traits at first because they simply have not paid enough attention to be able to notice them. Others may have less difficulty thinking of positive traits about themselves but may have trouble writing about it or talking about it. They often see it as bragging when it is not.

If any of those things apply to you, keep in mind to stay open when completing this exercise. The next worksheet will help you realize what good traits you have that you don't acknowledge often. When someone is used to giving all their attention to their negative qualities, they become comfortable in focusing on those only. Start asking yourself questions. Do you think it's fair to only focus on your negative traits? Would you judge your loved ones in the same way that you judge yourself? By visually being able to see what your positive traits are and beginning to acknowledge them, you start to move the rock in achieving a fair self-evaluation.

Worksheet #6.2

Documenting Your Positive Traits

What is the most common technique that people use to help remember things? Writing them down of course! If we must remember multiple things, we often create lists. This exercise is just like that. To begin learning how to acknowledge your positive traits, you will need to write them down in order to remember them.

How did you feel at the start of these worksheets when you were asked to write down your positive attributes? What emotions were you feeling? Anxiety? Uneasiness? Shame? Fear maybe? Did you start to think "I don't have anything to write!" or "What is there even to write?!" You need to start paying attention when these thoughts occur. Listen to those negative thoughts that pass through your mind when you are evaluating yourself. You may be showcasing a tendency to minimize your successes and maximize your failures. If you catch this happening, simply just acknowledge those negative thoughts, and let them pass without giving much weight to it. If those negative judgments keep occurring during your exercises, try writing them down. By writing these things down, it makes it easier for you to see how unfair those judgments are.

You are now ready to begin writing down your positive traits. The idea behind this is to create a list that contains all your positive qualities. This can include your talents, strengths, achievements, and personality traits. You can choose to record this in your own journal or write it down in this worksheet.

Here are a couple of tips you can keep in mind:

1. When starting these types of exercises, make sure you are scheduling a time in your calendar where you can give it all your attention. Don't do this while you are doing other things like watching TV or commuting. Give it the undivided attention it deserves.

2. Write down your positive attributes in your journal or on the worksheet physically. Don't just write it on scrap paper or make a mental note of it. This helps prevent you from losing your work when you want to look back on it.

3. Write as many positive traits that come to mind. There is no limit and definitely not "too many". Brainstorm as many as possible and you can add to it over the next few days until you've got a long list.

4. If you feel stuck, ask for help from a friend or family member. Ideally, this is someone that is supporting you throughout your journey of boosting self-esteem. Other people may be able to identify positive traits that you didn't know you had.

5. Pay attention to negative self-judgments that arise during this exercise. Naturally, people remember negative traits more than they remember positive traits about themselves. Remember that the positive traits you identify don't need to have been expressed 100% of the time. For example, if you wrote down that you are "disciplined" as a positive trait, but you took a day off

to rest from your projects last week, that still counts. Be fair in your own judgments.

6. Remember to look over the things you have written down in this exercise in the future. Don't just complete it and move on, it is important to look back on your work and reflect on the things you have written. This way it will help these positive traits sink into your mind and help you believe them.

If you find that you are having trouble thinking of traits, you can utilize these questions to help you:

- What is something that I look about myself?
- What are the positive characteristics that I have?
- What have I achieved in my life so far?
- What are some challenges that I was able to overcome?
- What are some of my skills?
- What have other people said about me that are positive?
- What are some qualities that I like in other people that I also share?
- If someone had similar qualities to me, would they be someone that I like?
- What are some qualities that I think are bad? Do I have any of these qualities?

To assist you even further, I have provided you a list of example positive characteristics.

Resourceful
Considerate
Strong
Organized/Reliable
Artistic
Avid Reader

Good-humored
Appreciative
Good Listener
Health Conscious
Friendly
Creative
Adventurous
Well-traveled
Praise Others
Diligent
Responsible
Politically Conscious
Fun
Animal Lover
Active
Charitable
Outdoors Person
Animal Lover
Loved
Good Cook
Cultured
Determined
Helpful
A Good Friend
House Proud
Movie Buff

Your Positive Traits Record

1. ____
2. ____
3. ____
4. ____
5. ____

6. ____

7. ____

8. ____

9. ____

10. ____

11. ____

12. ____

13. ____

14. ____

15. ____

16. ____

17. ____

18. ____

19. ____

20. ____

21. ____

22. ____

23. ____

Step 2: Affirm Yourself

People have a natural tendency to behave in accordance with their self-image. The technique of implementing change that lasts is to change the way someone perceives themselves. So how does affirmation play a role here? Affirmations are the valuable and uplifting assurances that we tell ourselves. These are very effective when used out loud so you are able to hear it from your voice. Humans naturally believe the things they tell themselves. For example, if someone hates something about the way they look, they will believe that they are an unattractive person. The next time you are in front of a mirror, practice affirmation by saying something you like about yourself.

As someone who is trying to increase their self-esteem, the affirmations they make should be focused solely on the positive things. If their affirmations are goal-related it will be best for them to act according to their positive personal values and their positive self-identity. This exercise below is built to help you build your own affirmations. Try to practice them frequently. This will aid you in building a positive self-narrative that helps increase your self-esteem over time.

Worksheet #6.3

Designing My Own Affirmations

This worksheet is split into two segments. The first is a step-by-step guide aimed to teach you how to design positive affirmations that you can repeat to yourself long term. Use these suggestions below to help make your own affirmations.

Part 1:

Tip	Example
Structure your affirmation "I statement". Start your sentences with "I am..."	I am a disciplined and hardworking player on this soccer team.
Focus on creating affirmations that have a positive outcome. Try to avoid using avoidant words such as "not" in your statements.	I am getting better at shooting goals after every single practice session.
Keep your affirmations as	I am appreciative of my

concise as you can.	amazing coach who is always helping me.
Design your affirmations to be as specific as possible, especially if it guides you to your goal.	I am more than qualified to get into this elite soccer team that I've been training hard for.
Try to write your affirmation in the present tense. Focus on using a gerund (a word that ends with "ing")	I am confidently improving my soccer techniques after every training practice.
Use descriptive words to give your affirmation more impact.	I am going to score at least 6 goals by next month.
Make your affirmations your own. They are personal and will relate to your particular goals rather than others.	I am impressing players on the other team by my good soccer technique.

Part 2:

Write down your affirmations in your notebook or in the lines below.

My Positive Affirmations

____

____

____

____

____

____

____

____

____

____

____

____

____

____

____

____

____

____

____

____

____

____

Once you have completed your positive affirmations, schedule a block of time every day or a couple times per week to look back at them and update them. The more you read them and drill them into your memory, the more positive thoughts will naturally come to you. You can also document any changes you feel in yourself as you do this exercise.

The next worksheet we are going to do in order to help more with your affirmations is less of an exercise but more of a guide. You will be doing something called the Mirror Technique. The concept here is very straightforward, you simply look at yourself in a mirror while saying the positive affirmations you wrote down to yourself. I know this sounds a bit crazy but the theory here is that by doing this, you are actually manipulating your subconscious mind to feel more confident.

Worksheet #6.4

The Mirror Technique Guide

The only tool you need for this exercise is a mirror. Start the exercise by standing in front of the mirror with a confident posture. Make sure your shoulders are rolled back, you are standing straight and your chin is pointed upwards. Look at yourself in the eyes and begin to repeat the affirmations that you've created for yourself. If you are able to do this daily, you will be impacted hugely. The only other thing you need is to have affirmations already prepared that you can use at every practice.

If you are looking to achieve maximum results, do this exercise twice a day. The most effective time to do this is in the morning right after you wake up and at night before you go to bed. By doing this in the morning, you will set a positive tone for the rest of your day. Your mind is also more impressionable in the morning and will aid your subconscious to take in the affirmations quicker and more deeply. Practice this once more before you go to sleep so those affirmations are the last things you think about before you fall asleep. Start easy and do it for two minutes at a time and try to increase it to 10 minutes when you have more experience.

Follow this step-by-step guide:

1. Stand directly in front of your mirror. Make sure your upper body is visible.

2. Make sure that your posture is good (shoulders rolled back, back is straight, chin tilted up slightly). Puff out your chest a little to make this easier.
3. Look into your own eyes and take a breath.
4. Repeat the first affirmation you wrote down about yourself. Go through the list of affirmations that you've written prior to this.
5. Read through your list until it runs out.
6. Repeat it again from the beginning until your two minutes is up (2 minutes for beginners and increase it by 1 minute every time you feel ready)
7. Allow yourself to absorb those words and let go of any negative thoughts you have of yourself.

Some people feel the results of this technique straight away while others need a few practices. Track your progress or just simply pay attention to the benefits you are receiving. Below is a checklist that I've written to help you identify some benefits you have gained.

- ❏ You begin to feel comfortable in your own skin.
- ❏ You are beginning to feel more accepting of your physical appearance.
- ❏ You notice an improvement in your communication skills.
- ❏ You are giving yourself an internal motivation boost before you do an activity.
- ❏ You are feeling more positive.
- ❏ You are starting to believe in your own capabilities and you feel like you are ready to try new things.
- ❏ You begin to feel less inferior to others.

❑ You are beginning to feel appreciation for yourself.

❑ You are starting to recognize your good attributes.

❑ You are no longer fearful of eye contact as before.

❑ You are starting to feel more confident when around other people.

❑ You are beginning to have a more positive opinion of yourself.

❑ You are being less doubtful about your ability and yourself in general.

❑ You are feeling more confident in your decision-making skills.

❑ You are setting higher goals and feel more confident about your ability to achieve them.

❑ You are starting to look and feel stronger.

❑ You are noticing that people are treating you differently.

Keep using this technique until you have checked off almost everything on this list. Some people believe that this technique is airy-fairy but try to actually believe the positive benefits you can gain when you say your affirmations out loud. The theory behind this technique is a combination of psychology, science, positive thinking, and hypnosis.

Step 3: Do Something That Scares You Every Day!

Often, people with low self-esteem are fearful of failure. Their fear prevents them from talking to new people or trying new things. The ideal method to overcome fear is to tackle it head-on. By just doing one thing that scares you every single day, you are gaining a multitude of experience and confidence. This exercise is something that increases a person's self-confidence significantly.

Everyone has felt the dread before doing something they are intimidated by. Those with low self-esteem feel this more often than others. Practicing doing scary things every day no matter how significant or insignificant, will make everything in general, less scary. They will be able to build resilience towards fear. In this step, we will be completing a worksheet where you write down the things you are afraid of and how and when you will face it head-on.

Worksheet #6.5

Exercise: Do One Thing That Scares You Everyday

The most difficult part of this exercise is figuring out where to begin. Don't worry, below is a detailed example of which you can base your own off while creating your personalized plan.

Example:

My Fear:	What action I will do to conquer my fear:	When I will do it:
I have a fear of strangers talking to me when I am out in public.	The next time I am using public transit I will greet someone I don't know with "Good afternoon!" or "Happy Friday!"	Tomorrow afternoon when I am taking the subway to get home from work.
I have a fear of bumping into people I know when I go to a popular coffee shop.	The next time I run into a person I know I will simply say hello. If conversation ensues, I will try to engage.	The next time I run into someone at the coffee shop. Likely on Saturday mornings.
I am afraid of rejection if I ask my crush out on a date.	I will start a conversation with my crush by simply greeting them. I will suggest a casual outing like a coffee or lunch to chat with them more. I will keep in mind that rejection is alright and that it is not a bad thing. I will go in with the mindset that either answer they	Next Thursday afternoon I will greet my crush and ask her out on a date.

	give me is acceptable.	
I am afraid of social outings with my coworkers.	The next time a coworker suggests an outing, I will not turn it down and accept the invitation. I will try my best to get to know them better.	Next Thursday when Sarah suggests going out for happy hour.
I am afraid of looking stupid if I ask questions during a work meeting.	I will purposely find a good question to ask in the next work meeting. For example; "Mr./Mrs. Manager, what are your thoughts on this change?"	I will do this the next time a meeting is scheduled.
I am afraid of embarrassing myself in public like spilling something in front of people.	I will purposely spill something slightly in public, not on myself, but outside on the ground. I will take on other people's reactions. It probably is not as bad as I think it is. They will likely not remember this.	I will do this on Saturday morning.

By writing these fears down I am hoping that you will realize how silly some of these fears seem to be. When you take the initiative to face your fears, you may realize that you dealt with it so easily that it was silly of you to have these fears in the first place. By conquering fears, you will naturally gain confidence and doing this every day will help boost your self-esteem. Below is a worksheet where you can write down the things that you are afraid of, how you are going to overcome them, and when you will do it.

My Fear:	What I will do to conquer my fear:	When I will do it:

When you start this exercise, start to record your findings in the following worksheet (worksheet #6.6). By keeping a record of how you feel after facing each fear you can look back on it and see your progress. This is useful when you must face larger fears in life and during those hard times, you can look back on this to give yourself the confidence that you can overcome that fear too.

Worksheet #6.6

Fears That I Have Overcome:	How I Feel About This Fear Now:
Ex: Asking my crush out on a date.	*My fear of asking people out has shrunk. I felt horrified when I first asked my crush out on a date but when she responded so casually with a "yes!", I began to feel more comfortable with asking people out.*

Use this checklist below to keep track of the benefits you are starting to gain by doing these fear overcoming practices.

❏ You are beginning to realize all your potential as a person.

❑ You are beginning to accept that instead of running away from your fears, you are practicing ways to overcome them so it gets easier every time.

❑ You are starting to realize that being afraid is a waste of energy.

❑ You are beginning to realize that fear is all in your mind.

Step 4: Question Your Inner-Critic

The next step in this 10-step journey is to question your own inner-critic. Individuals who have low self-esteem often have very active and inaccurate inner critics. Therapies such as Cognitive Behavioral Therapy (CBT) is effective in helping people learn to start questioning what their inner critic is saying to them rather than just listening to it and accepting it. For instance, if an individual finds themselves thinking that they are useless, they will begin to question their critics by saying "What evidence is there that supports the accusation that I am a loser?" and "What evidence is there that doesn't support the accusation that I am a loser?" People often find that there isn't much or any evidence that supports the negative statement that their inner critic said about them. The ability to catch themselves thinking of thoughts without supporting evidence is a sign that you have learned to question your inner critic.

In this step, we will be focusing on catching the times where our inner critic begins to say negative things about ourselves and then find a way to contradict those statements. Before we begin, look at this list of responses you can say in response to your inner critic.

1. Stop saying the same negative statements about me. I have supporting evidence that I am not any of those things you are describing me as. I will change you, so you begin to tell me more encouraging things instead.

2. You are lying. I have evidence that does not support the statements you are saying about me. I've taken an objective look at myself and I am not the things you are saying.

3. I belong. You are mimicking the voice of the bullies in my childhood and your words are false. I have grown up to be a respectful and good person.

4. I am not weak. I have faced and conquered so many of my fears and I plan on facing more of them. Your words do not have any supporting evidence.

5. I am not scared. I have faced my fear head-on and conquered them. I will continue to do this.

6. Stop beating me up. Stop hurting my esteem just because I don't want to have more negative thoughts. I will replace your negative words with positive thoughts about myself and my goals.

Worksheet #6.7

Training Your Inner Critic (Four-Step Guide)

Step 1: Revive Your Curiosity

The first you need to take in order to tame your inner critic is to simply just be aware of it. By being aware of it, you will need to be curious. Most people in modern-day society move through their lives in a passive manner. Due to how fast-paced things have become nowadays if we don't give our thoughts and feelings the attention it needs, we tend to forget about them. Even though everybody feels numerous emotions daily, they don't acknowledge them every time. Instead, people have learned to simply react to everything and turn on auto-pilot. When we do this, we don't question or evaluate the downsides to the actions and decisions we are making.

Living on autopilot is the easiest option for a lot of people. Due to the number of decisions people need to make in a day, living on autopilot means that they can avoid making those decisions. People have learned to just accept how things are even if we dislike them. We'd rather not spend the energy or effort in changing things. However, if you are reading this book, I think it's safe to say that you do want to change your life and you are not happy with where it is at. You are actively making decisions and taking actions to work on your self-esteem, self-confidence and managing your inner critic. The first step that you need to take in this process is to simply just be more curious about the thoughts that occur in your mind. Try to ignite some curiosity regarding your emotional experiences and pay attention to the way you speak to yourself when you are in a conflict or approached by a challenge. This may sound like it's easy but acknowledging your passive thoughts is actually hard since we are so used to living on autopilot. Our minds automatically filter out certain things all since it knows that you don't like to think about it.

Here is the first exercise in this process. Below is a list of questions that you will use to question your inner critic. You can do this in planned sessions or you can keep these questions handy and ask your inner critic when it is awake. This decision is entirely up to you but just make sure you are doing this as it will make the later exercises more effective.

1. What is my Inner Critic saying to me?
   A:____

   ____

   ____

____

____

2. What is my Inner-Critic saying about me specifically?

   A:____

   ____

   ____

   ____

   ____

3. When does my Inner-Critic say these things? Be as specific as possible.

   A:____

   ____

   ____

   ____

   ____

4. As a result of those things, what do I normally think about myself?

   A:____

   ____

   ____

   ____

   ____

5. What are the common patterns and themes that I recognize regarding my inner critic?

   A:____

   ____

   ____

   ____

   ____

6. How do all these things together affect my overall behavior?

   A:____

   ____

   ____

   ____

   ____

7. What do all these thoughts say about me?

   A:____

   ____

   ____

   ____

   ____

8. Where do these opinions come from?

   A:____

   ____

   ____

   ____

   ____

9. Are these opinions factual or are they all made up?

   A:____

   ____

   ____

   ____

   ____

10. Is it even appropriate to think this way in this certain situation?

   A:____

   ____

   ____

____

____

11. Where/when did I start learning to think this way?
    A:____

    ____

    ____

    ____

    ____

12. Are there any childhood experiences that stand out to
    me? Do I think that these experiences influence the
    way I think now?
    A:____

    ____

    ____

    ____

    ____

13. Is there anybody that may have instilled these thoughts
    into my mind?
    A:____

    ____

    ____

    ____

    ____

14. Does this type of thinking even make sense, logically?
    A:____

    ____

    ____

    ____

    ____

When you answer those questions, you are actually helping yourself analyze the progression of your thoughts and what role they play in real-life situations. You are now able to see the relationship between past experiences and if it is affecting the way you behave now.

Step 2: Acknowledge Your Inner Critic
Rather than falling back into old habits of ignoring or rejecting your inner critic, we will practice acknowledging it instead. People often resist thinking about a certain thing but they just end up thinking about it more and end up having a larger effect on their life. Rather than resisting this step, acknowledge the words of your inner critic instead. Try shifting your mind and think of your inner critic's words as opinions and concerns for your well-being rather than insults. Try to believe that your inner critic has the best intentions for you and is trying to help you. Although it may be hindering right now, your inner critic actually comes from a place of concern and care. In the following exercise, start having a conversation with your inner critic and them ask them the following questions. Write down your answers in the lines below.

1. What is my inner critic trying to protect me from?
    A:____

    ____

    ____

    ____

    ____

2. What does my inner critic not want me to feel or experience?
    A:____

    ____

    ____

____

____

3. Why is this important to my inner critic?
   A:____

   ____

   ____

   ____

   ____

4. Are the words my inner critic is using critical or
   constructive?
   A:____

   ____

   ____

   ____

   ____

5. Are the words being used designed to help me improve
   or to criticize me?
   A:____

   ____

   ____

   ____

   ____

6. Are the words being used based on factual evidence?
   Or are they based on an opinion?
   A:____

   ____

   ____

   ____

   ____

7. If I take these words into consideration, where in my life might I need to make some changes?

A:____

____

____

____

____

8. How else could I make changes in my life without all this resistance from my inner critic?

A:____

____

____

____

____

When you finish this exercise, remember while moving forward that your inner critic is a part of you. It is a part of you in the way that a worried parent or friend wants to look out for you and is trying to protect you from any harm. However, your inner critic is actually biased because it comes from a place of wanting to protect you so their positive intentions are holding you back from personal growth. Ultimately, it is crucial for you to know the differences between your inner critic's protection from your actual capabilities.

Step 3: Thank and Appreciate Your Inner-Critic

In step 3, we will take the time to thank our inner critics for their constant concern and them for always wanting to jump in and help out. Your inner critic has shared numerous opinions with you and now it's time to interrupt them and change the way they are helping you to something you can actually benefit from. If the things your inner critic is saying has justification, then you can go ahead and listen to it for guidance. However, if it doesn't have justification, then it's safe to say that their suggestions are empty. In this exercise, we will be thanking our inner critic for everything they've done. Fill in the blanks below.

Dear Inner-Critic,

Thank you for always cautioning me of _______________________________. Thank you for always watching over me in _________________ situations. I appreciate all the different times that you told me that I can't do _________________, but I want to tell you that I am capable of doing ___________. Instead of telling me lies that you have heard from my childhood, or other people in my life, I want you to tell me constructive criticism such as; ___________. You are always welcome to give me feedback but if you are acting stubborn, I will ignore you.

Sincerely,

____

Step 4: Negotiate with Your Inner-Critic

The ideal situation is to come to a mutual understanding with our inner critic. Remember that the primary concern of your inner critic is your safety. They want to keep you away from harm and therefore, instead of just ignoring your inner critic find a way to prove to them that why the decisions you are making are out of best interest for yourself. It is possible that your inner critic will give way and give you an easier time to pursue the things you want.

In this exercise, you will be filling out the chart below. This chart will help you identify the things your inner critic is saying to you and what you can say to negotiate with it. I have provided you with a few examples to give you a better understanding.

Your Goal	What You Expect Your Inner-Critic to Say	How You Will Negotiate with Your Inner-Critic
Ex: I want to get another college degree so I can learn a new skill that will help me get a job in that field.	*Ex: You have already been working full time for three years, by going back to college now you are admitting to others that you have failed your career. People will judge you.*	*Ex: Not everybody will like me so judgments from others are normal. I am not happy at my current job so starting something new is healthy for me. My happiness and wellbeing are more important than the things people might say about me.*
Ex: I am hating my job right now and I want to quit to travel the world for a few months.	*Ex: Quitting a full-time job is an irresponsible thing to do. You just want to take a long vacation. You will never accomplish anything if you quit.*	*Ex: I am not a quitter as I have seen many things throughout my life. I don't want to keep working a dead-end job that I'm miserable in. Traveling is not the same as an extended vacation, I want to learn new things about the world.*

Step 5: Do the 100 Days of Rejection Challenge

Give yourself a pat on the back for making it this far into the guide. You have probably realized many things about yourself at this point. This step is the hardest step in the entire guide. We will be doing the 100 days of rejection challenge. It is exactly what it sounds like. The idea of this challenge is to make outrageous requests of other people knowing full well that they will reject you. The purpose of this is to help desensitize rejection so you are no longer fearful of it. This way, you will learn to be able to ask for what you need or want no longer fearing the possible rejection.

Worksheet #6.8

100 Days of Rejection Challenge

This challenge is simple. Over the next 100 days (about 3 months), you will be asking one person a day, a request that is totally crazy. You will allow them to reject you and you will do this 100 times until you feel desensitized from the answer "no". This may sound intimidating but the outcome is entirely worth it. You could make this more fun by asking a friend or a loved one to join you in this challenge. Some people take this challenge to another level by making a blog/vlog or sharing it with social media. This way, you will have some encouragement and fun along the way.

Below is the worksheet that you will be filling out over the next 100 days. There are a few examples provided for you but get creative with your own.

- ❏ Challenge #1: *Ask a stranger to loan you $100.*
- ❏ Challenge #2: *Ask the barista to give you free coffee.*

❏ Challenge #2: _______________________
❏ Challenge #_: _______________________
❏ Challenge #_: _______________________
❏ Challenge #_: _______________________
❏ Challenge #_: _______________________
❏ Challenge #_: _______________________
❏ Challenge #_: _______________________
❏ Challenge #_: _______________________
❏ Challenge #_: _______________________
❏ Challenge #_: _______________________
❏ Challenge #_: _______________________
❏ Challenge #_: _______________________
❏ Challenge #_: _______________________
❏ Challenge #_: _______________________
❏ Challenge #_: _______________________
❏ Challenge #_: _______________________
❏ Challenge #_: _______________________
❏ Challenge #_: _______________________
❏ Challenge #_: _______________________
❏ Challenge #_: _______________________
❏ Challenge #_: _______________________
❏ Challenge #_: _______________________
❏ Challenge #_: _______________________
❏ Challenge #_: _______________________
❏ Challenge #_: _______________________
❏ Challenge #_: _______________________
❏ Challenge #_: _______________________
❏ Challenge #_: _______________________
❏ Challenge #_: _______________________
❏ Challenge #_: _______________________

❑ Challenge #_: _______________________
❑ Challenge #_: _______________________
❑ Challenge #_: _______________________
❑ Challenge #_: _______________________
❑ Challenge #_: _______________________
❑ Challenge #_: _______________________
❑ Challenge #_: _______________________
❑ Challenge #_: _______________________
❑ Challenge #_: _______________________
❑ Challenge #_: _______________________
❑ Challenge #_: _______________________
❑ Challenge #_: _______________________
❑ Challenge #_: _______________________
❑ Challenge #_: _______________________
❑ Challenge #_: _______________________
❑ Challenge #_: _______________________
❑ Challenge #_: _______________________
❑ Challenge #_: _______________________
❑ Challenge #_: _______________________
❑ Challenge #_: _______________________
❑ Challenge #_: _______________________
❑ Challenge #_: _______________________
❑ Challenge #_: _______________________
❑ Challenge #_: _______________________
❑ Challenge #_: _______________________
❑ Challenge #_: _______________________
❑ Challenge #_: _______________________
❑ Challenge #_: _______________________
❑ Challenge #_: _______________________
❑ Challenge #_: _______________________
❑ Challenge #_: _______________________

❏ Challenge #_: _______________________

❏ Challenge #_: _______________________

❏ Challenge #_: _______________________

❏ Challenge #_: _______________________

❏ Challenge #_: _______________________

❏ Challenge #_: _______________________

❏ Challenge #_: _______________________

❏ Challenge #_: _______________________

❏ Challenge #_: _______________________

❏ Challenge #_: _______________________

❏ Challenge #_: _______________________

❏ Challenge #_: _______________________

❏ Challenge #_: _______________________

❏ Challenge #_: _______________________

❏ Challenge #_: _______________________

❏ Challenge #_: _______________________

❏ Challenge #_: _______________________

❏ Challenge #_: _______________________

❏ Challenge #_: _______________________

❏ Challenge #_: _______________________

❏ Challenge #_: _______________________

❏ Challenge #_: _______________________

❏ Challenge #_: _______________________

❏ Challenge #_: _______________________

❏ Challenge #_: _______________________

❏ Challenge #_: _______________________

Step 6: Set Yourself Up for Success

Self-esteem often suffers when a person becomes discouraged about their abilities when they fail to achieve their goal. This will happen frequently if this person is always setting very difficult goals. If the purpose is to increase their self-esteem, start setting more reasonable goals that can be achieved more easily. Rather than a person setting one huge goal like "I want to buy a vacation house by the end of this year" they can break the big goal into smaller ones such as "I want to see a financial advisor to see how much money I need to save in order for me to be able to buy a vacation house."

When a person has found success from achieving small goals, they begin to feel good about their accomplishments, therefore, having the confidence and experience to tackle bigger and harder goals. The key to this technique is to document all of their achievements as a reminder to themselves all the things that they have succeeded.

To-Do lists are very helpful for many people in everyday life; however, people don't tend to look back on them to remind themselves of the things they've accomplished. By being able to look back on past accomplishments, you can remind yourself to feel proud of the things you've done. This helps build confidence.

In this worksheet, we will be focusing on breaking down bigger goals into smaller and more achievable ones. There will be two different lists, the first one focuses on the large goals and the second one focuses on smaller goals. This exercise will guide you so you can see what the smaller steps are that you can take in order to make your way to accomplishing a larger goal. By tracking your progress, you can build confidence and get the inspiration needed to continue pursuing your goals.

Worksheet #6.9

Building Small Goals Out of Big Goals

Big Goals:	Smaller Goals Made from Big Goals:
Ex: I want to purchase my first vehicle by next year.	*I will re-do my budget to save $200 a week, amounting to $800 a month.* *I will do research every week to find the best sales and deals on new cars (e.g. Black Friday, Boxing Day...etc.)* *In six months, I will have enough for a $4,800 down payment.*
Ex: I want to become a licensed electrician.	*By the end of the month, I will have completed all the research on electrician schools in my area.* *I will begin to study every week until applications are open.* *I will submit at least 4 applications to a few*

	different schools when applications begin. *When I get into school, I will start to look for part-time work to get more hands-on experience.* *Once I graduate, I will study to pass my certification.* *Once I get my certification, I will apply to at least two full-time jobs per week.*

In this example you can see how building smaller goals out of your big goal gives you a more detailed look into the things you need to do. It helps a big goal feel more manageable and real. By accomplishing those smaller goals, you are giving yourself small wins throughout the process that leads to a big win. Try to direct your energy to your smaller goals that relate to your big goal, try to accomplish that set before jumping onto another set of smaller goals. Stay committed and concentrated, this will help you accomplish goals much more efficiently.

Step 7: Help Other People

We talked about how helping other people is an effective way to boost self-esteem in the previous chapters. By helping others, it helps us shift our attention and focus away from ourselves to someone else. Helping others helps us feel grateful for the things that we have and it feels good to be able to make a difference for someone using your skills. Focusing on yourself is good especially when you are trying to grow your self-esteem but helping other people will help your self-esteem grow as well.

According to scientific research, when people help others, the portion of their brain that is responsible for joyful and rewarding feelings becomes activated. That area of the brain that is activated releases the hormones that make us feel good.

What are some ways that you could help others? The simplest and most straightforward way is to just start volunteering in your community. It could be working with children, the homeless or even just at your local library. This is a good way of gaining some perspective of people that are less fortunate. Often, some of the things that people are upset with not having, or the constant comparing to others, is immediately gone when you spend some time experiencing how less fortunate people get by. Certain things that people used to be upset about becomes trivial when they gain a new perspective. Here are a few questions to consider when it comes to helping others:

- Do I like being around children, the elderly, or animals?
- How much of my time am I able to offer to others?
- What belongings do I have and no longer need that someone else can benefit from having?

- What skills do I have that local non-profits in my city could use?
- Do I have the financial resources to donate to a nonprofit of my choice?
- What am I generally interested in?

The way you help others doesn't have to be a grand gesture. You can do something very simple like paying it forward. You can simply leave behind a few dollars for the next person at your local drive-thru or coffee shop. This will make the day for the next person in line. Or you can just take a friend or family member out for dinner for no reason. There are so many little nice things that you can do for others that will help increase your self-esteem.

Worksheet #6.10

Helping Others

In this exercise, you will be writing down people that you could help and what things they may need help with. After that, you will follow up with an idea of how you can help them. The purpose of this exercise is to help you brainstorm some ideas that you can take action on. By keeping this list around, you can slowly do these things over a period and give yourself a boost of self-esteem here and there. Helping people also creates good dialogue which leads to building potential friendships. Shift your focus yourself to other people every now and then so you can help increase your sense of purpose.

Someone That Is in Need:	What I Can Do to Help Them:
Ex: My coworker has been struggling to pay her bills recently and has only been eating fast food for lunch.	*I will bring some of my leftover home-cooked meals for her to eat for lunch. I'll bring it into work so she can have at least one healthy meal a day.*

When you finish these exercises, try to document your feelings and the reactions of those that you helped. Try to notice if you feel different after helping someone. You can keep a journal to document your thoughts and feelings after completing acts of kindness. By writing your feelings down, it helps them feel more real.

Step 8: Self-Care

Learning to take care of yourself is the only feasible way to have good emotional, physical, and social health. It is hard for anyone to feel good about themselves if they constantly don't feel healthy or feel good about their physique. Try to make time for exercise and get into a habit of sleeping at healthy times and opt for healthier food options. Try to avoid unhealthy things like going to bed late at night and waking up in the afternoon the next day - these things tend to make people feel unproductive and lazy. Instead, try to get a quick exercise in when you wake up in the morning to get your juices flowing. This can be something very simple like 20 push-ups and 20 sit-ups. Moreover, start opting for healthier options when you eat your meals. Avoid fast food or eating out if you can and get into the habit of buying fresh foods and making it yourself. This makes a huge difference in your health. By staying away from packaged and processed foods, your overall health will improve.

Let's begin learning about various ways that someone can increase their self-esteem by practicing self-care. Below are a few recommendations that you can utilize. Try to make an effort to do at least one thing from this list every day, consistency is the key to making a good change.

1. Read a book at the end of your day to wind down rather than watching TV or browsing your phone. Reading helps get your brain going and is actually scientifically proven to be more fulfilling than watching television.
2. Get as much fresh air as you can. Try to take some time every day to go outside for a run or a brisk walk. Pay attention to the beauty of your surroundings when you are outside.

3. Buy yourself a nice meal at a restaurant you like. The thought of eating alone may seem scary at first but it is very relaxing and gives you the opportunity to really taste and appreciate your food.

4. Listen to music more often. When people are busy, they tend to forget about the existence of music. Make a playlist of all your favorite songs and just listen to them when you have free time.

5. Add one healthy thing to your daily routine. This could be choosing to walk a part of your daily commute or walking up the stairs rather than getting on an elevator. Do something that gets your blood flowing.

6. Nurture your body by doing something easy like putting on a face mask or drawing yourself a bath. If you have the money for it, book yourself a massage or facial. Doing this more often helps you feel taken care of.

7. Start a new exercise routine that is achievable. Like we talked about earlier, making a 5-minute routine in the morning when you wake up helps you feel energized for the rest of the day.

8. Awaken your inner child by doing something that you loved as a kid. This could be drawing, riding a bike, or swimming. Try to get back into your old hobbies to ignite some of that joy.

9. Turn your phone on silent more often. Set a time in your day where you set your phone to do not disturb so you can't get work calls or anything of that sort. Spend more of your free time having face to face connections with people.

10. Try to laugh more often. If you are choosing to spend some time watching TV or a movie, choose something fun that can incite some laughter. Laughing is a great way for your brain to release some endorphins.

Worksheet #6.11

Self-Care Checklist

This exercise is different from the previous ones. I will be providing you with multiple self-care items that you will have to do one every day to help you take better care of yourself. Often, people have trouble finding things that they can do to take care of themselves. This exercise will give you numerous different self-care tasks that you can do at a minimal cost.

Choose one self-care task from below and try to do one every day, fill in the date that you have completed it on.

Self-Care Task	Its Benefits:	Date Completed:
Cooking meals at home using fresh ingredients avoiding processed foods. Find a simple recipe online to follow to make this easier.	Cooking helps create feelings of confidence and fulfillment. Healthy meals are nourishing for the body and will help a person feel better overall.	
Incorporate a session of exercise every day, no matter how short or long. This could be going to the gym	Getting exercise helps get people's juices flowing which helps them feel healthier overall. It will make them feel more confident in their	

or just doing a quick stretch or push-ups in the morning.	physique.	
Draw a bubble bath when you get home from a long day.	Warm baths are very effective in releasing tension from the body and is also a great way to practice mindfulness.	
Read one chapter of a book of your choice before going to bed.	Reading is a much more fulfilling task than watching television. This will give the person a quick self-esteem boost.	
Book a massage or facial appointment on the weekend.	Massages are a great way to relax your body and mind. People often feel refreshed and tension-free after a massage.	
Treat yourself to your favorite restaurant. Go alone and give your attention to the food and atmosphere.	Eating alone is a great way to get a new perspective on dining out. The person will be able to taste their food better and enjoy some alone time.	
Go out for a stroll at sunset.	Sunsets are breathtakingly	

	beautiful. By going out for a walk during this time, you will be able to get some exercise while getting to see one of the most beautiful things in this world.	
Organize one spot in your home.	Clutter is often responsible for making people feel stressed and anxious. Choose one spot in your home to organize, this will make a person feel more relaxed.	
Stay hydrated	Being properly hydrated makes the world of a difference in a person. Feeling healthier helps a person feel more confident. Make sure to be drinking the recommended amount of water per day for your body type.	

Do an assessment once you have completed a few of these self-care actions. Have you noticed any change in your self-esteem? Do you feel more confident after completing certain actions? Keep a note of these changes that you can use as inspiration to keep up with these habits.

Step 9: Set Boundaries

Having personal boundaries is important in order to maintain high self-esteem. The ability to say no and telling others to respect your boundaries is very important especially if you are someone who often commits to too many things. Individuals with low self-esteem have the most trouble saying no because they want to prove their worth by doing things for other people. Boundaries are a crucial part of building respectful relationships. Boundaries are responsible for the limits of acceptable behavior for the people in your life. They are what protects you from others taking advantage of you or putting you down.

If you are someone that often feels uncomfortable with the way other people are treating you, it is a sign that you need to set personal boundaries and make it known to others. People with weak boundaries often are taken for granted and are in vulnerable positions. By creating strong and healthy boundaries, you are telling people that you need to be treated with respect. This is what protects people from getting into relationships with those who will take advantage of their goodheartedness.

Worksheet #6.12

Setting Strong Boundaries

If you are someone that feels like people are often crossing your boundaries, it is time to reset and strengthen them. Start by writing down in the space below an experience where an important person or a loved one has made you feel hurt or unhappy.

____

____

After this, try to think about what the other person's intention was. Were they putting you down to try to make themselves feel better? Were they trying to take advantage of you? Were they trying to make their own lives easier by asking you for help?

Then, decide what you would like to do next. For instance, if your sister is taking advantage of your generosity by always borrowing your car, you can write down "I understand that you don't have a lot of money so you'd rather drive my car than to call an Uber, but could you start asking other people so it's not always my car that's being borrowed?" You can put a positive spin on it and add at the end of your statement "You know that I am more than happy to help you but I'm just asking to have my car back more often than not so I can use it for my own things." In the space below, write down a response you would say to someone who crosses your boundaries next time.

Remember how important it is to be able to say no when people are asking unreasonable things of you. It is totally fine to also reject reasonable requests every now and then if they conflict with your schedule. Moreover, if you notice that people around you mask their insults to you with humor, don't be afraid to challenge them. You can say something on the lines of "I don't think what you said was very funny and it can actually be very hurtful if I had taken it the wrong way!" Remember that you are not crossing other people's boundaries so make sure you are not insulting anyone by masking it with humor.

The next thing you are going to do is to fill in the list below with the things you'd like people to stop doing to you, around you, or saying to you.

5 Things I'd Like People to Stop Doing Around Me
Ex: Stop cracking race jokes around me or stop criticizing people that aren't around to defend themselves.

1. ____
   ____
   ____

2. ____
   ____
   ____

3. ____
   ____
   ____

4. ____
   ____
   ____

5. ____
   ____
   ____

Give Things I'd Like People to Stop Doing to Me
Ex: Stop borrowing my things without asking or stop blasting music at home when I am trying to sleep.

1. ____
____
____

2. ____
____
____

3. ____
____
____

4. ____
____
____

5. ____
____
____

Five Things I'd Like People to Not Say to Me
Ex: Don't apply to that job, you don't qualify for it anyway or you're never going to succeed!

1. ____
____
____

2. ____
____
____

3. ____
____
____

4. ____

____

____

5. ____

____

____

Next, look at what your current boundaries are and ask yourself the questions below. Write your answers down in the lines provided.

- How much attention do people expect from me at a moment's notice?

____

- Do you always make yourself available when somebody needs you? (e.g. do you answer your phone no matter what you are doing?)

____

- How often do you receive praise and acceptance from others?

____

- What is the reason that you are popular with your friends? (e.g. Do they genuinely like you? Or did they start giving you attention once they realized you had something they needed?)

____

- How and what do you feel after spending time with your friends or family? (e.g. Do you feel drained? Do you feel fulfilled?)

____

When people grow, their boundaries stay the same so it requires updating if their life is changing. They may have been able to offer more time to their friends and family in a previous time in their life but may become much more limited if they had started a new job or is in a relationship. By updating boundaries, it doesn't mean that a person no longer wants to help other people anymore, it just means that they want to be able to keep some time for themselves too. Remember that the act of resetting boundaries does not guarantee that the people around you are going to be supportive of that change. More often than not, some people may become very resistant to it because they liked the old ways of doing things. Be prepared that some people may lash out to you or say hurtful words like "you've changed" to showcase their disapproval at the new boundaries. Keep in mind that just like everything else in life, changing things may come with a price. This can cause you to lose some friends or peers along the way but that just means that those relationships would not have survived in the long term anyway. Here are several tips to help you deal with people's disapproval when it comes to your new boundaries:

- Be adamant with your new boundaries no matter what persuasions are being thrown at you. (e.g. Don't flex your boundaries just because someone said "Just one more time!")
- Keep your boundaries concise and easy to follow (e.g. I'm turning off my work emails after 6 pm on weeknights)
- Always remain calm !
- Don't blame others for your emotional reactions, instead, be responsible for them.
- If a situation comes that may require compromising, be flexible. Do what makes sense for you but don't agree to anything that doesn't feel okay to you.

When you have reset your boundaries to something that is more updated, stronger, and clearer, respectful people will be accepting of them. By doing this, it means that you can now be yourself and ask for the things you want and need. This will shield you from potential manipulators in your life.

Step 10: Shift Your Mentality to Equality

In the final step of this guide, we will be focusing on adjusting our mindsets to one that is founded upon equality. People with low self-esteem often see others are more worthy or more deserving than them. Rather than keeping this unhealthy perception, it is important for them to try to see themselves as equals.

In the present day, people of the minority often face prejudice like sexism and racism. If you are of a minority group, you may struggle feeling equal when you are surrounded by people that have the privilege. You feel that you must work harder than other people to achieve the same recognition. This may be a harsh truth in today's society but your mindset still has to be that you ARE equal to other people. It is alright to put in the extra work in order to prove yourself but you have to understand that you don't NEED to do it.

Chapter 7: How to Use Self-Acceptance to Improve Your Self-Esteem

At this point in the book, we are going to introduce the concept of self-acceptance. It can be defined in three different ways:

1) Self-acceptance is the feeling of being satisfied with yourself despite your past choices or behaviors
2) Self-acceptance is being aware of your strengths and weaknesses
3) Self-acceptance is having a realistic assessment of your capabilities, talents, and overall worth

In summary of those three definitions, self-acceptance is the happiness and satisfaction that you have with yourself that is needed to achieve good mental health. Having self-acceptance means that you are able to understand who you are, be realistic about it, and be aware of what strengths and weaknesses you have. Those who have high levels of self-acceptance tend to also have a more positive attitude, do not wish to be different from who they are, accept all traits of themselves, and are not confused with their identity.

You may be wondering how all of this relates to self-esteem? Well, self-esteem is defined as having confidence in your own ability and self-worth and self-acceptance is being aware and satisfied with all your strengths and weaknesses. Self-acceptance does not need to rely on achievement to make one feel worthy. It makes people feel worthy by simply being comfortable and happy with who they are.

So, how does self-acceptance work in the real world? Based on scientific studies, self-acceptance has 5 different stages. The first stage is the Aversion. People's natural response to uncomfortable feelings or situation is either avoidance or resistance. For instance, if somebody dislikes a trait that they have, it is natural that they avoid it rather than dealing with it head-on. The second stage is curiosity. When aversion no longer works, people will become curious to learn more about their problems. This curiosity is the driving factor behind people looking to learn more about their problems. The more curious a person is, the more likely they are to have a fulfilling life. People who lack this curiosity tend to shy away from problems leading to get stuck in stage one which is aversion. The third stage is tolerance. Those in this stage will wish that their problems will go away while enduring it the entire time. Many people in this stage still suffer the effects of their problems but are forcing themselves to tolerate it so they can go on with their everyday life. The fourth stage is allowing. As people's resistance slowly drains away, they then allow themselves to feel. Rather than just recognizing and tolerating, they acknowledge them and feel the emotions that occur. This is the stage of acceptance where they accept their problem and allows themselves to feel all the emotions that come with it. The fifth and last stage is friendship. During this, people begin to see the value that their feelings bring and decide to accept them rather than willing them to leave. They become comfortable enough to be friends with those feelings regardless if it's good or bad.

Examples of Self-Acceptance

In this subchapter, we will be exploring some examples of self-acceptance in practice. Those who have mastered the art of self-acceptance can look at themselves in the mirror and accept 100% of who they are. They no longer try to ignore, fix, or explain any faults or flaws that they think they have.

Self-acceptance is different for everybody. It heavily depends on the struggles that a person has gone through and what parts of their lives that they'd rather not look at. Right below are a few examples of what other people's self-acceptance looks like:

- A person that is in the process of divorce feels like they have failed in life. However, this person experiences self-acceptance by realizing that they have made mistakes in their life and their marriage has failed but it does not make them a complete failure.
- A person suffering from bulimia may accept themselves as a person with an imperfect body or perception but is committed to changing their perspective.
- A student who studies really hard in college only to get mediocre marks can reach the point of self-acceptance where they realize that test-taking and studying may not be their strength, but this is okay because they have other strengths that they can build on.
- A person with low self-esteem who avoids acknowledging their self-deprecating beliefs may experience self-acceptance by first acknowledging them and realizing that not every single thought that they have is necessarily true.
- A worker who is having trouble meeting the goals set by their unreasonable boss might accept themselves by accepting the fact that there will be times where they won't be able to deliver on unreasonable timelines. However, they are still a good person, even if they couldn't deliver on time.

Hopefully, you were able to see the pattern in these examples. Self-acceptance is the act of realizing that although you may not be perfect in all aspects of your life, it doesn't mean that you are completely invaluable. By having self-acceptance, you are giving yourself permission to be bad at certain things but also giving recognition to the things you are good at. For a person to have healthy self-esteem, they must learn to be self-accepting and to let go of any negative judgments they have for themselves.

Using Self-Acceptance in Therapy

One of the largest uses of practicing self-acceptance is its huge role in therapy. Research has found evidence that people who lack self-acceptance tend to also have lower levels of happiness and well-being. They often are found to have disorders like anxiety and depression. If the theory is that low self-acceptance causes low mental wellbeing, it means that high levels of self-acceptance can act as a protective factor against bad mental health. The concept of self-acceptance being the foundation of good wellbeing is the reason why self-acceptance is often incorporated into therapy.

If you have ever been to therapy, you are likely to have learned about the importance of accepting yourself and your reality. It is likely that your therapist has taught you to acknowledge all traits (good and bad) and learn to accept them. Keep in mind that self-acceptance is about the ability to accept yourself fully and it doesn't mean that you are excusing any harmful or bad behavior. It is important that you are able to accept the truth that you have engaged in bad actions previously and you do have undesirable traits but these are all the things that are part of being you.

This distinction is really important to make because people get confused about needing to accept themselves if they have done something awful. Accepting reality does not mean you condone it or that you like it. In the same way, accepting yourself does not mean you have to celebrate and like every part of yourself. Be able to accept the not so positive things about you is a crucial step in improving and adapting.

At the end of this chapter, you will be given multiple worksheets that will aid you in achieving self-acceptance. These are suitable for those who want to boost their self-esteem or are battling more serious problems like addiction.

Using Self-Acceptance for Addiction Recovery

Self-acceptance is often used to help the people that are recovering from addiction. This is extremely important to those people who abuse substances as they often use coping mechanisms like denial to avoid coming to terms with their problems. They often use unhealthy habits like minimizing, forgetting, rationalizing, lying, or even repressing to not face their problem. Although these coping methods can be helpful in certain circumstances, it is not a practical solution if they are trying to recover.

When an addict comes to terms with their problem, they often think that they need to control every single aspect of their life because they want to recover. This is not a healthy mindset to be in because there are numerous things in our lives that we cannot control.

This is why self-acceptance is so important in all kinds of recovery processes. Before being able to make a change in your life, people who struggle with addiction have to accept the following:

- The reality that they have a problem.
- The reality that it's impossible to control every aspect of their life.
- The reality that everyone has flaws just like them.
- The harsh reality of their situation.

When a person is able to accept the reality of who they are in the moment, they can start to work on changing the aspects within their control. The idea behind this is not to promote self-blame but to change their mindset to "Who I am right now is someone I don't like and I am going to help myself change this." By giving yourself an opportunity to change is one of the powers of self-acceptance. By doing this you will be fully grounded in your reality and choose to help yourself out of it rather than criticizing yourself.

Self-Acceptance Worksheet Exercises

In this chapter, we will be focusing on worksheets that will help you build self-acceptance. It is crucial that you work on these as self-acceptances is one of the cornerstones to building healthy self-esteem.

Worksheet #7.1

How Would You Treat A Friend?

The purpose of this exercise is to help you initiate compassion for yourself by treating yourself the way you would treat a friend. It's easier to be loving and forgiving to friends and family but it is much harder to extend that same kindness to ourselves. This exercise is simple, read the questions below and write down your answers to them.

1. Think back to a time where you had a good friend or a family member that felt down about themselves and was struggling. What was your response to your friend during this situation? Please write down what you would say and what tone you would say it in.

____

____

____

____

____

2. Now think back to sometimes where you would feel badly about yourself. What is your response to yourself during these situations? Write down what you would say to yourself and the tone you would say it in.

____

____

____

____

____

3. Is there a difference between the above two situations? If there is, why is that? What factors come to mind that may lead you to treat yourself differently than the way you treat others?

____

____

____

____

____

4. Write down possible things that would change if you had treated yourself the same way that you would be treating someone else during a time of hardship.

____

____

____

____

____

Worksheet #7.2

Self-Compassion Bank

In this exercise, we are going to be focusing on improving your understanding of yourself and the love that you have for yourself. This exercise just requires a few minutes of your day where you focus on showing yourself compassion.

Let's begin by thinking about a past situation in your life that has caused you stress or anxiety. Tap into that situation and see if you can feel the actual discomfort of anxiety and stress in your body.

Start to say to yourself:

"This moment is one of suffering." or "This is stressful." or "This is hurting."

Then, say to yourself:

"I am not alone." or "Other people feel this way too." or "Suffering will always be a part of life."

Now, place your hand over your heart and feel the warmth and the gentle touch of your hand against your chest.

Say to yourself:

"May I be kind to myself."

Feel free to take this exercise one step further and ask yourself "What are the things that I need to hear right now in order to express kindness to myself?" Here are some examples:

"May I find strength."
"May I offer myself patience."
"May I offer myself the compassion that I need."
"May I offer myself forgiveness."
"May I accept myself for who I am."

Worksheet #7.3

Using Writing to Find Self-Compassion

Those who enjoy writing or prefer to express themselves using words will find this exercise very helpful. This worksheet is set up into three segments and is also effective for people who aren't writers.

Follow these directions below:

Part 1:
Start by thinking about all the weaknesses you have that cause you to feel inferior. Everybody has various things that they may not like about themselves or makes them feel unequal.

Next, think about things that make you insecure. If there is one particular item that stands out to you, bring it to the forefront of your mind.

Pay attention to your feelings when focus on your insecurity. Notice what emotions and feelings arise and let yourself experience them. People often disallow themselves to feel negative emotions but these are all important parts of life. Negative feelings can also bring out positive outcomes such as self-acceptance.

Simply feel those emotions that arise while thinking about your insecurities. Write a blurb on the emotions that you feel:

____

____

____

____

____

____

Part 2:

Now that you have written about your emotions, you can begin the second part of this exercise. In this exercise, you will be writing a letter to yourself from the perspective of a sympathetic loved one or imaginary friend.

The purpose of this exercise is to show you the compassion and understanding that you often to show to your friends, to yourself.

Start this exercise by imagining a friend who is a compassionate, kind, accepting and unconditionally loving person. Then, imagine that they share the same strengths and weaknesses as you.

Think about how this friend would think about you. They love you, they are kind to you, and they accept you. Even if you have done something to hurt their feelings, this friend is understanding and is quick to forgive.

Your friend is understanding and sympathetic but they also know everything about your life. They know every decision that you've made to get to where you are, each step that you took in your journey, and they acknowledge all the factors that have played a role in who you are today.

Next, write a letter to yourself from the perspective of your imaginary friend. Tailor the body of this letter on the insecurities that you have written down in part one. Think about the things this friend would say to you.

Will they tell you that your mistakes and weaknesses are unacceptable? Will they tell you that you need to be perfect? Or will they tell you that they sympathize with all the feelings you are going through?

Would they be mad at you if you feel inadequate or insecure? Will they happily encourage you to accept everything about yourself? Will they remind you of your positive traits and your strengths?

Write this letter in their perspective and make sure you are showcasing themes of kindness, compassion, and love.

Dear __________,

____

____

____

____

____

____

____

____

____

____

____

____

____

____

____

____

____

____

____

____

____

____

____

Sincerely,

____

Part 3:

When you complete this letter, take a short break, and give yourself some space away from this exercise.

When you are ready to come back, read the letter you wrote with the intention to really take in what it's saying. Don't just read it as something you wrote for yourself but read it as if it really were from a friend.

Open yourself up to the sympathy and compassion that your friend is showing you. Let those words comfort and soothe you. Let those words sink in and have it turn into compassion for yourself.

Worksheet #7.4

Inner Critic Job Description

This practice is here to help those who are often battling with their inner critic. This exercise is meant to aid those who simply just agree and give in to the opinions of their inner critic. By completing this exercise, it will help people understand the true responsibility of their inner critic. Follow these instructions below:

In this exercise, you will be writing a job description for your inner critic. Your inner critic has held this job for all your life, it is time to get an idea of what their main responsibilities, skills, duties, and qualifications are.

The responsibilities of your inner critic are the primary purpose of its existence. For instance, your inner-critic's responsibilities are to keep you safe and comfortable for as long as they can. They are also responsible for motivating you and punishing you to keep you in line.

Your inner critic's duties are the specific ways they go about doing things in order to try to fulfill their responsibilities. For instance, if your inner-critics responsibility is to keep you safe and comfortable, it could mean that they may be telling you to avoid getting close with other people in order to prevent heartbreak.

Your inner-critic's skills and qualifications are the things that make them good at their job. For example, utilizing humor to mask your insecurity or vulnerability or speaking loudly so they end up at the forefront of your mind.

There will be no right or wrong answer in this worksheet. The goal here is to simply understand all the reasons why your inner critic is here and what its actual job is.

Your Inner-Critic's Job Responsibilities

1. ____
   ____

2. ____
   ____

3. ____
   ____

4. ____
   ____

5. ____
   ____

Your Inner-Critic's Job Duties

1. ____
   ____

2. ____
   ____

3. ____
   ____

4. ____
   ____

5. ____
   ____

Your Inner-Critic's Skills and Qualifications

1. ____
   ____
2. ____
   ____
3. ____
   ____
4. ____
   ____
5. ____
   ____

Follow Up Questions:

- Does your inner-critic's main responsibility line up with your own values?

  ____
  ____

- How successful is your inner critic at meeting the responsibilities?

  ____
  ____

- How much energy does it require to complete this job?

  ____
  ____

- Are there any other skills that would help out your inner critic?

  ____
  ____

Worksheet #7.5

Compassion Focused Therapy (CFT)

The following worksheet is more of a guide than an exercise. This guide is here to help you learn about compassion focused therapy and how it can play an important role in our lives. This is something you want to read if you are having difficulty expressing compassion to yourself.

Let's start by learning some of the background information on CFT:

- CFT was developed to help manage feelings of self-loathing, criticism, and shame.
- CFT is useful when treating mental illnesses or other related problems.
- CFT is founded on a new model that was built from the science that backs human nature, attachment, and evolution.

Now, let's talk about how evolution has shaped the human brain.

- There are three layers in our brain, each being more modern than the last:
  - Reptilian Brain: The oldest and most basic part of our brain, its focuses are survival, territory, food, and temperature.
  - Mammalian brain: The next level up from the reptilian brain, it is focused on living with groups, nurturing, status, and hierarchy.
  - Human brain: This is the most modern development of the brain and is focused on caregiving, relationship forming, and higher-order thinking.

The CFT model is explained by the following:
- The CFT model proposes that humans use three systems to manage their emotions:
    - Threat System: The motivation behind this system is to survive and its attention is focused on the fight or flight mindset, threat, fear, anxiety, and danger.
    - Drive system: The motivation behind this system is to win and its focus is on goals and finding an advantage.
    - Caregiving system: The motivation behind this system is to look after and soothe another, its focus is other's distress or pain.
    - Everyone is born with all these systems ready to go. Depending on our environment, it determines which systems are used.

Since compassion helps manage the symptoms of mental illness:
- The goal of CFT is to help people utilize and further develop their caregiving system. This is what will help them come to terms with their thoughts and feel comfortable in their own bodies.
- The caregiving system aids in activating warmth, empathy, strength, kindness, non-judgment, wisdom, and moral courage.
- The practice of CFT is divided into three parts:
    - Learning the skills needed to develop the caregiving system
    - Learning about human nature
    - Practice activating the caregiving system and implementing it in daily life

Here are some key messages to keep in mind:
- "The bad things that have happened in your life are not your fault. However, you will be the one that is responsible for alleviating your own suffering."
- "Compassion is all about choosing to be the best version of yourself."

Next, we are going to learn about the process of forming compassion for yourself. Don't be intimidated although it seems like a hard process because of how deeply out self-criticism is embedded within us, and how long it's been there for.

The CFT follows this format "Problem > Coping Strategy > Unintended Consequences". It focuses on the importance of compassion.

The first step here is to figure out all the past influences that lead you to feel self-criticism and shame in the present day. This step here helps you acknowledge these shameful memories or past trauma that may have manifested into shame.

In the space below, write down the fears you struggle with the most. Give attention to the feelings of blame, criticism, and shame. Keep in mind that there are two types of fear, internal and external. Internal fears are like depression, anxiety, rage, or shame and external fears could be when someone hurts your feelings.

____
____
____
____
____

Next, write down some defensive measures that you have in place to avoid getting hurt or to lower the risk of getting hurt. This could be avoiding social contact altogether as a way to prevent rejection.

____

____

____

____

____

Internal defensive behaviors are often used by people to keep themselves from feeling those difficult emotions or problems. This includes things like dissociating, substance abuse, self-harm, or a constant reminder of weaknesses. External behaviors are used to avoid being harmed by other people. This includes being silent, submissive, and keeping a distance from other people.

In the last exercise here, we will learn about the effects of the cycle of safety and defensive behaviors that relate to unintended consequences. These consequences are the outcomes from the safety behaviors that a person exhibits although they may not be intending to produce them. These consequences can be self-harassment or emotional isolation. In the space below, write down what sort of safety behavior you think you have and write down whether you think it is harming you or protecting you.

____

____

____

____

____

These unintended consequences likely have a large impact on how you understand yourself. People may attack themselves for exhibiting these unintended consequences which may spiral into even more unhealthy defensive behaviors. This cycle tends to feed on itself.

This worksheet is often emotionally difficult to complete because you have to dig deep and find out that you haven't shown yourself enough compassion. This is an important step for those working on their compassion and self-acceptance to identify these bad behaviors and begin to change them.

Worksheet #7.6

Changing Your Inner-Critic Self Talk

This worksheet is meant to be completed over the next several weeks. It will eventually form the map for the way that you will be changing how you relate to yourself in the future. Certain people find it useful to negotiate with their inner critic through the act of journaling while others find it more helpful to negotiate using internal dialogue. If you are somebody who prefers to write, journaling is a great way to take on this transformation. If you are someone who does not like writing all too much than the internal dialogue method will work just fine. Feel free to speak to yourself out loud or think quietly.

1. The first step you need to take in order to change the way you think and treat yourself is to pay attention to the moments where you are being self-critical. There may be a situation where your inner critic has something negative to say, and this happens so often that you don't notice it anymore when it happens. During the moments where you are feeling down, think about what your inner critic has said to you. Be as specific as possible and pay attention to the exact

words that were being used. What words were they? Are there specific statements that are used more commonly than others? What was the tone of your inner critic's voice? Was it mean? Angry? Harsh? Does its voice remind you of things that people in your past have said to you? You want to reach a point in your self-awareness where you understand your inner critic so well that you've become aware when it begins to say something. For example, if you skipped a class today, does your inner critic say "you always skip class" or "you are so careless". Get a detailed idea of what your inner critic says to you.

2. Put in the effort to try to soften the tone of your inner critic. Don't say things like "I hate you!" but instead say something like "I understand where you are coming from and I know that you are worried about me getting hurt. However, the things you are saying are unhealthy. Could you let me compassion say a few things to you to help you understand a bit better?"

3. Reframe the observations that were made by your inner critic into something that is more positive. If you are struggling to come up with words to rephrase it with, think back to what your imaginary compassionate friend would say to you in that situation. It is more helpful to use endearing terms especially those that express care and warmth. For instance, you could say "I understand that you skipped class today because you were feeling very upset and you think staying home will make things better. However, it seems like now you feel even worse so why don't you try to go outside for a little bit and see if that makes you feel better?"

Worksheet #7.7

Self-Compassion Journal

This exercise utilizes writing and journaling to express your emotions. This has been proven to be effective in improving a person's mental wellbeing. When you have a few moments to sit back and review how your day went, use this journal to write down the things you felt negative about, things you've judged yourself for, or any painful situations that you endured. For instance, the waitress that was serving your lunch today messed up your order and you lashed out at her out of frustration. Afterward, you felt very embarrassed and guilty about it. For these events, practice using mindfulness, kindness, and a sense of common humanity to help yourself process events in a more compassionate manner.

1. Mindfulness: This is the act of bringing your awareness to the emotions that arose during your difficult situation. Write down how you felt in that situation. When you are writing, don't be judgmental of what happened but try to accept it as the way it is. Don't make it dramatic or belittle it.

2. Common Humanity: This is the act of thinking about how your experiences are related to a larger human experience. This will require you to acknowledge that imperfection comes with being human and everybody has had similar painful experiences. Remember the different conditions and causes that a painful situation has underlying. For instance, my frustration at the waitress was more extreme than usual because my boss yelled at me all morning. I was already in a bad mood and that one event tipped me over the edge. If it weren't

for how badly my day started, my reaction would have been different.

3. Self-Kindness: This is where you will write down words that are kind, understanding, and comforting for yourself. Tell yourself that you do care and that you are trying to learn a way to speak to yourself that is gentler. For instance, say things like "It's okay. I know I was really rude to the waitress, but I can understand where my frustration came from. I will return to the restaurant tomorrow and apologize and leave her a good tip."

By practicing using these three components of compassion, you will learn how to acknowledge your thoughts and also be able to look back on them in a more positive way. By upkeeping this journal, you will be practicing self-compassion which will eventually become stronger and is more easily applied in your life.

Chapter 8: The Importance of Self-Awareness

The next thing we need to learn is self-awareness. What exactly is it? In its simplest terms, self-awareness is the ability to be aware of the 'self'. The self is the thing that creates and maintains our unique identity. Experiences, thoughts, and abilities are all the components that make it unique. Self-awareness was studied first back in 1972. Researchers that studied this concluded that when people focus their attention on their inner selves, they are able to evaluate their behavior against the standards and values that they hold for themselves. They become conscious of themselves and are objective evaluators of their own actions. The conclusion that the researchers came to has become the current foundation of self-awareness.

One thing to keep in mind is that self-awareness is not only about noticing the things within ourselves, but it is also about how we see our inner world. For instance, everyone has at least judged themselves once on the thoughts or experiences they've had. However, it is important to be able to have a non-judgmental reflection of oneself. So, if the act of being non-judgmental is a component of self-awareness, how does one begin to achieve that? When people notice the things happening inside of them, they are able to acknowledge and accept it as a part of being human. People should be doing more accepting rather than beating themselves up for mistakes that are inevitable.

Self-awareness also goes way beyond just having knowledge about ourselves. It is also about paying attention to our wellbeing by having an open mind. The human mind is exceptional when it comes to storing information and memories and begins to form the blueprint of our emotional life. This information ends up coaching our mind to react in similar ways when similar situations arise. Self-awareness helps us to be aware of this conditioning which will free our minds from unhealthy habits.

Self-awareness is one of the most important components in achieving high emotional intelligence. This is an aspect that is important to everybody regardless of how much self-esteem they have. Emotional intelligence is a person's ability to monitor and control their thoughts and feelings. Those who have higher emotional intelligence have the ability to act more consciously rather than passively. They tend to have better mental health and a positive outlook on life. In addition, these people have wider and deeper life experience and are likely to be a more compassionate person. A scientific study recently studied the components of self-awareness and found that insight, mindfulness, and self-reflection are all aspects of self-awareness and can bring benefits such as having less emotional burden and becoming someone who is more accepting. This research also found evidence that supported self-awareness as a critical trait for those who strive to be successful business leaders.

At this point, you may be wondering why self-awareness is not a more prominent trait within humans when it's such a crucial concept to our wellbeing. The answer to this is that people are generally just not observing themselves as often as they should. They don't pay attention to the things that are going on inside and outside of them. Most people nowadays live their lives on autopilot where they don't pay attention to what they are doing and what emotions they are feeling. They let their minds wander to other things that aren't the things that are happening in the present moment.

If a person is constantly mind-wandering, it is a symptom that they are lacking self-awareness. This symptom affects people's ability to get a good and accurate understanding of who they are which then leads to a higher likelihood that they will believe the things that their inner critic tells them. For instance, if an individual strongly believed that they are a loyal friend, then they are more likely to interpret events where they made mistakes as an anomaly of their identity which is a 'loyal friend'. This pre-existing belief influences people regarding how they handle aftermaths of situations. If the individual in that example accidentally forgot about a gathering they were supposed to go to with their friends, they are likely to just brush it off as a one-off accident since they have the perception of themselves that they are a 'loyal friend'.

How Will Self-Awareness Benefit Me?

Just like we are discussing this now, the value that self-awareness brings has been researched and discussed by numerous psychology experts and professors. Most of them noted that the main benefit that self-awareness brings is the ability for a person to see themselves clearly, understand who they are, and how other people perceive them. Self-reflection is the tool that is needed for a person to examine themselves and attain self-awareness. It is a conscious and deliberate method that helps people grasp a better understanding of their thoughts, emotions, and experiences. This also includes the ability to understand how other people see them.

Here are some benefits of self-awareness:
- Improves people's critical-thinking and decision-making skills.
- People gain better listening skills and empathy due to enriching their emotional intelligence.
- People enhance their skills that are related to leadership.
- People will enhance their communication skills which leads to strengthening relationships.

People who have increased self-awareness make for better team players and employees. According to statistics, people who have more self-awareness are recorded to be less likely to cheat, steal, or lie. Self-awareness isn't only beneficial to those that are looking to boost their self-esteem, but it is beneficial to many employers that look to hire people who can bring productivity, engagement, trust, company culture, and better employee communication.

In the world today, there is a growing understanding that self-awareness is one of the key driving components of leadership skills. Good leadership skills are the differentiating factor from good performance to great performance.

There are two main types of self-awareness that we have to keep in mind. The first type is the traditional internal self-awareness and it refers to how a person views and understands their inner self. The second type is external self-awareness which is the ability to understand how other people see them. Those who are able to have the most benefits of self-awareness are the ones that are able to achieve both types.

How Does Self-Awareness Relate to Self-Esteem and Self-Acceptance?

If self-awareness is the ability to be aware of who you are and self-esteem is the way a person perceives themselves and how they judge their actions and thoughts then they work hand in hand because self-awareness is something a person needs to achieve in order to be able to change their self-esteem. If a person isn't able to recognize who they are or what their achievements are, it will be really hard to change the way they see themselves.

By improving and developing one's self-awareness, they will be able to tap into important things such as their inner-critic and have the ability to change the negative opinions they hear into something more constructive. The ability to speak kindly and positively to yourself helps increase a person's self-esteem.

These three components of self-awareness, self-esteem, and self-acceptance all rely heavily on one another to build the healthiest and happiest version of oneself. Self-awareness allows a person to realize who they are and self-acceptance is the ability to accept everything a person is regardless of good or bad. Self-esteem is a combination of those things and acts as the lens that a person looks through to see themselves. By lacking either one of those components, a person's inner self becomes unbalanced which then takes a negative toll on their mental wellbeing.

Chapter 9: Self-Esteem Exercises

In the final chapter of this book, you are provided with additional worksheets that you can use to help you reach your goals. These worksheets range from topics like increasing gratitude all the way to exercises that will further help you build self-esteem. You don't need to complete all these exercises if you don't want to since you have already completed the core exercises throughout this book, but if you are looking to get some extra reinforcement, this chapter will be useful to you.

Worksheet #9.1

Exercise: Increasing Gratitude

This worksheet contains multiple exercises that focus on increasing gratitude. The purpose of this is to do exercises that will help a person increase their level of gratitude. Increasing gratitude helps individuals can feel more positive emotions that are associated with having greater happiness. The ability to be thankful for the things one has in life will help people shift their mindset away from the constant need to want things.

Exercise #1: Journal About Gratitude

Take a few minutes every morning or before you go to bed to write down five good things that happened in your day. Keep in mind that it doesn't have to be a major event (like winning a prize from a lottery ticket) but it can be simple things like having a good meal, the nice weather, or just having a good chat with a friend. Be as consistent as you can with this journal as only doing it occasionally won't be effective compared to doing this multiple times a week. Write down your gratitude in the lines below.

____

____

____

____

____

____

____

____

Exercise #2: Write A Letter

In this exercise, try to think of a person who has been a major impact on your life. This could be someone that you really appreciate having in your life or just someone you'd like to thank. Then, write them a letter containing the specific details regarding the things you appreciate about them and mail it to them. Follow the guide below to create a quick draft of the letter. Use pen and paper to write the actual letter as it indicates more sincerity compared to a typed letter.

Who:

____

____

What they did to impact me:

____

____

What I am thankful for:

____

____

Exercise #3: Visit Someone That You Appreciate

This exercise is similar to the one you did above. You will write a letter to someone else that you appreciate but instead of mailing this letter, deliver it in person instead. Try to keep this letter a surprise by not telling the person why you are visiting. You can even read them the letter and then give it to them for keeping. Many people may be skeptical of this exercise but it has been proven to be extremely effective due to the gratitude that the receivers get from reading a kind letter.

Exercise #4: Take A Gratitude Walk

Go for a walk in your local neighborhood and try to absorb and appreciate your surroundings. Try to notice things that you normally don't pay attention to like the buildings around you, the smell of the air, or the nature around you. Spend a few minutes during your walk to solely focus in on each of your senses (sight, touch, taste, smell and hearing). Try to look for new things during your walk in your everyday environment that you normally don't pay attention to. Write down some new appreciations that you may have discovered through this walk and how it affected your mood.

____

____

____

____

____

Worksheet #9.2

Self-Esteem Journal

The purpose of this exercise is to use a journal to document the good and positive things that you did throughout the week. You will also include the positive emotions that you feel when you witness other people accomplishing things. Use the outline below and fill out this journal throughout the week in order to remind yourself of what you are capable of.

Monday	Something great that I did today...	
	I had fun when...	
	I felt proud when...	
Tuesday	Today I completed...	
	I had a good experience with...	
	I did some things for other people...	
Wednesday	I felt great about myself when...	
	I felt proud of someone else when...	
	Today was an interesting day because...	

Thursday	I felt proud of myself when...	
	A good thing I witnessed was...	
	Today I accomplished...	
Friday	Something great that I did today...	
	I had a good experience with...	
	I felt proud of someone else when...	
Saturday	I had fun today when...	
	I did this for someone today...	
	I felt great about myself when...	
Sunday	A positive thing I saw today was...	
	I had an interesting day because...	
	I felt proud of myself when...	

Worksheet #9.3

Exploring My Strengths

People who have the self-awareness to recognize and understand their strengths often use those strengths more frequently which leads to them having more areas of success in their life. These people often feel happier, are more likely to succeed in their goals and have higher self-esteem. The ability to recognize and use your strengths is due to the process of understanding what those strengths are and how a person can use them. Some strengths are easier to recognize than others. Harder strengths to recognize are the ones that feel normal to a person even though it may not be a strength that is commonly had.

In this exercise, you will be identifying your strengths and the ways that you are currently using them. You will also find new ways to utilize your existing strengths to your advantage.

Circle your strengths out of the list below and add your own strengths in the bottom row.

Optimism	Independence	Flexibility	Adventurousness
Wisdom	Artistic Ability	Curiosity	Leadership
Athleticism	Discipline	Assertiveness	Logic
Empathy	Honesty	Open-Mindedness	Persistence

Ambition	Creativity	Confidence	Intelligence
Enthusiasm	Love of Learning	Love	Social Awareness
Gratitude	Kindness	Cooperation	Spirituality
Fairness	Bravery	Humor	Forgiveness
Modesty	Common Sense	Self-Control	Patience

Relationships (romantic, friendships and family)

List the strengths that you have that help you within your relationships.

____

____

____

____

____

Describe a time where your strengths helped you in a relationship.

____

____

____

____

____

Describe two new ways that you could utilize your strengths within relationships.

1. _______________________________

____

____

____

____

2. _______________________________

____

____

____

____

Profession (Present or past work, professional endeavors, or school)

List the strengths you possess that help you within your profession.

____

____

____

____

____

____

Describe a time (be specific) that your strengths have helped you within your profession.

____

____

____

____

____

____

Describe two new ways that you could utilize your strengths within your professional life.

1. _______________________________________

2. _______________________________________

Personal Fulfillment (interests, hobbies, extracurricular activities)

List the strengths that you have that help you achieve personal fulfillment.

____

Describe a time (be specific) where your strengths were able to help you within personal fulfillment.

____

Describe two new ways that you could use your strengths for personal fulfillment.

1. ____

____

____

____

____

2. ____

____

____

____

____

Worksheet #9.4

Challenging Your Negative Thoughts

Negative thoughts created by your inner critic often result in low self-esteem, depression, and anxiety. A person who constantly receives positive feedback on what they do can still feel like they are awful at their job due to one criticism. Irrational thoughts about a person's overall performance in life often dictates how they feel about themselves. Practicing challenging these thoughts help people begin to change them into ones that are more positive.

Answer the following questions:

Is there significant evidence for my thoughts?

____

____

____

____

____

Is there evidence contradicting my thoughts?

____

____

____

____

____

____

Am I starting to interpret this situation without considering all evidence?

____

____

____

____

____

____

What would a friend or family member think about this situation?

____

____

____

____

____

____

If I look at this situation in a positive light, how is it different?

____

____

____

____

____

____

Will this situation matter one year from now? What about five years from now?

____

____

____

____

Worksheet #9.5

Identifying Your Core Beliefs

Each single person on this planet views the world through a different lens. Two people who have gone through the same exact situation could have different interpretations of it. The core beliefs that we have are the ones that we value deeply within us and influence how a person interprets their experience in life. You can think of your core beliefs like a pair of sunglasses. Everyone has a pair of them but everyone has a different lens shade that causes them to see the world in their own unique way.

Here is an example:

Situation	Core Belief	Consequence
You meet somebody new and you are thinking about asking them to go out for a drink.	I'm not worthy.	Thought: Why would this person want to go out for a drink with me? Reaction: You will not ask the person for a drink due to fear of rejection.
	I am worthy.	Thought: We might have a lot of fun if we had a drink together. Reaction: You will ask the person out for a drink

People who have negative core beliefs often are led to more harmful consequences. In order to begin challenging these beliefs, the person would need to identify what those beliefs are. Below are a few examples:

I'm a bad person	I'm abnormal	I'm undeserving
I'm unlovable	I'm stupid	I'm boring
I'm not good enough	I'm ugly	I'm worthless

List one of your negative core beliefs:

____

List three statements of evidence that contradicts your negative core belief.

1. ____

   ____

2. ____

   ____

3. ____

   ____

Worksheet #9.6

Self-Esteem Building: Sentence Completion

In this simple exercise, we will be doing sentence completions. This exercise is an easy and effective way to help remind ourselves of the positive attributes we have. All you have to do is to fill out the rest of these statements with the things that hold true to you.

I was really happy when...

____

____

____

Something that my friends like about me is...

____

____

____

Something that my family likes about me is...

____

____

____

I am proud of accomplishing...

____

____

____

My family was happy when I...

____

____

____

In school, I am good at...

____

____

____

At work, I am good at...

____

____

____

Something that makes me different is...

____

____

____

Worksheet #9.7

Positive Steps to Wellbeing

This last exercise in the book will simply be a quick guide to remind you of the things that you need to be doing on a daily and weekly basis in order to keep boosting your self-esteem and mental wellbeing. Post this guide up somewhere where you can see every day and make sure to be following it. It is easy to slip back into old habits and that is something that you don't want if you are set on making changes in your life.

Be Kind to Yourself	Exercise Regularly
Everyone is made up of different components like religion, genes, culture, gender, education,	Being active is crucial as it has the ability to lift our mood, reduces emotions like stress and anxiety, improve

upbringing, sexuality, life experiences, and beliefs. Everyone has bad days. Make sure to be kind to yourself and focus more on encouragement rather than criticism. Treat yourself with the kindness that you would treat a loved one in the same situation.	physical health, and simply just gives us more energy to do things. Try to spend more time outside, ideally somewhere with green space or near a body of water. Find an activity that is outside that you enjoy doing and do it.
Take Up A Hobby And/or Learn A New Skill Picking up new hobbies or learning a new skill is very helpful in increasing a person's confidence. It also helps build interest, gives you the ability to meet more people, and to prepare yourself for finding new jobs and career paths.	**Have Some Fun/Be Creative** This one is quite obvious, having fun and channeling some creativity is important to helping people feel better while increasing their confidence. Make sure you are trying to do fun things every week so you can enjoy yourself and get your mind away from negative thoughts.
Help Other People Try to get involved in an opportunity where you can help your community, project, charity, or just someone you know personally. Helping others will make you feel better	**Relax** Make sure that you are making time to care for yourself. Allow yourself to relax and chill and find something relaxing to do that suits you. Different people require different

about yourself as well as bringing benefits to others and enriching your own community.	things to relax. You can also practice some breathing exercises that can teach you to relax deeply.
Eat Healthy Eating regularly and incorporating lots of fruits and vegetables in your diet will help quick start your healthy diet. Make sure to eat breakfast, don't skip meals, and drink lots of water.	**Balance Sleep** Help yourself get into a healthy sleeping routine by going to bed and waking up at the same time every single day. Irregular sleeping habits are hard on a person's body and can cause negative side effects like drowsiness or anxiety.
Connect with Other People Humans are naturally social beings. Make sure you are staying in touch with your friends and family and that you are contacting them regularly just to talk or meet up face to face.	**Beware of Drugs and Alcohol** Avoid alcohol and drugs, especially if you are using it as a coping mechanism. These substances tend to have a depressive nature and tend to add to your problems rather than helping them.
See the Bigger Picture People give different meanings to different situations and often sees things from a point of view that is built by their beliefs	**Accepting** People often fight their negative thoughts and feelings in order not to deal with them. Instead, try to pay attention to them and

and upbringing. Try to widen your perspective and look at the bigger picture. Ask yourself questions like "Is this fact or opinion?" or "What meaning am I giving to this situation?" or "How will other people see this situation?" or "Is there another way to look at this situation?"

give up that struggle. Some situations are not within our control to change so you can accept them and move on rather than trying to change it or battling with it. Allow those battling thoughts and sensations to just be and they will naturally pass.

Conclusion

By the end of this book, you should be feeling like you have gotten a good understanding of the fundamentals of self-esteem and the components in your life that you would need to change in order to boost it. Just to recap, you have learned that self-esteem is not the same as self-confidence and what the fundamental differences are. You learned the importance of each and why they work hand in hand to enable a person to have a healthy mental wellbeing. You also explored the different causes of low self-esteem and how it typically starts in a person's childhood. After that, you explored all the different benefits that come with increasing a person's self-esteem. This was extremely important as understanding these benefits will become the driving factor behind all the hard work that you are going to do in order to increase your own self-esteem. Then, you explored all the benefits that come with improving self-confidence which in turn also helps you with self-esteem. After that, you explored an important chapter where you learned to identify what your level of self-esteem is. You learned that the self-esteem spectrum ranges from low self-esteem to high self-esteem with healthy self-esteem in the middle. You also learned those people with high self-esteem don't mean that they have healthy self-esteem and in fact, it is just a technique to cover up the fact that they have low self-esteem. The chapter after that was the important guide of 10 steps to help you start improving your self-esteem. You did various exercises throughout these 10 steps and this is likely the longest chapter you've had to work through. By the end of that chapter, you began to learn about other components of self-esteem like self-acceptance and self-awareness. These components play a big role in a person's ability to boost self-esteem as they all have a strong relationship with one another. Lastly, you were provided with a chapter that is just full of additional worksheets you can use to help gain more self-esteem. These are extremely important as it is easy to fall back into old habits if one does not continue to try in completing the practices for self-esteem.

Now that you have excellent knowledge of everything to do with self-esteem and how to increase it, what are the next steps? The short answer for you is consistency. You learned that self-esteem fluctuates depending on a person's circumstance. By continuing to remind yourself of how self-esteem works and continuing to do exercises even if you have healthy self-esteem will prevent it from fluctuating a lot when you are faced with an obstacle in life. We learned that it is silly to think that a person's journey through life would be smooth and obstacle-free. By continuing to practice exercises and completing worksheets to help build a more positive inner self, you are more well-equipped to handle obstacles on your own when they do arise.

One of the last messages that I want to get across to you is how important consistency is moving forward from this book. You are the only person that can hold you accountable to continue completing exercises and practicing the self-care needed to have a healthy self-esteem. In the last chapter of this book, I provided you with a quick guide in self-care that has a list of components that you should be doing every day in order to maintain a healthy lifestyle. By feeling healthy, positive, and energized, a person is more likely to feel good about themselves which is a great self-esteem boost. However, being stuck in unhealthy habits like eating badly, avoiding social contact, or sleeping irregularly are all habits that decrease a person's self-esteem. Remember that even someone who has always had healthy self-esteem is still at risk of having low self-esteem depending on their life situation, their outlook on the world and their ability to deal with problems. Nobody is 100% shielded from developing low self-esteem. The only thing you can do is to keep maintaining your self-esteem so there is a lower chance that an obstacle or situation in your life can bring you down.

The exercises throughout this book are designed to help anyone that is looking to grow or maintain their self-esteem. A common theme that I tried to emphasize throughout your journey is that simply doing these exercises once will not be helpful in the long run. For a person to see long term success, they are going to have to incorporate these exercises into their daily routine. For example, we went through an exercise where you wrote out in a chart a list of people that could use your help and what you were going to do to help them. Only doing that once during your assignment of the exercise will only provide short term benefits. However, if you incorporate helping someone every day or even every week, you are getting into the habit of doing good for your community and providing yourself with a sense of fulfillment. This holds true for all the other exercises that you are provided. When you get to the point where you have finished all the worksheets in this book, simply just start over from the beginning. Keep doing this until it becomes a habit and these exercises will simply become reinforcement for your self-esteem rather than a boost.

In conclusion, I'd like to thank you for taking the initiative in changing your life. The easier option is to just go along with how things have always been and find coping mechanisms to deal with unfortunate things that happen. Instead, you took the harder route and decided to find ways to change yourself into someone that you can be happy with. This doesn't mean that you are trying to accomplish more goals or become more successful. This simply means that you are beginning to practice being happy with who you are and accepting everything about yourself regardless of good or bad. Remember, self-esteem isn't about accomplishing more things so you can feel good about yourself, it is about changing the way you see yourself and the ability to a perception that is more positive. In turn, you will gain more confidence about your ability which will motivate you to try new things and pursue new goals. When you start doing that, that is when you will start seeing success in your life. As much as a low self-esteem can be a vicious cycle, having healthy self-esteem is a good cycle as accomplishing goals helps you build more self-esteem and having more self-esteem helps you work harder to achieve goals. So again, I'd like to thank you for taking the time to change your life for the better. Remember, if you feel like you've fallen off track, simply just pick up this book again and start from the beginning.